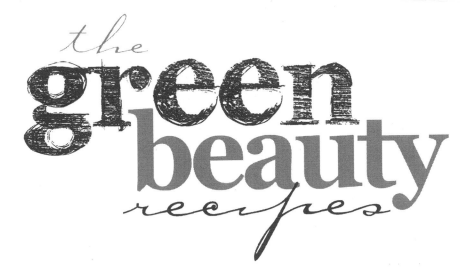

# the green beauty recipes

Easy Homemade Recipes to Make Your Own
Natural and Organic Skincare, Hair Care,
and Body Care Products

Julie Gabriel

# Green Beauty Recipes

Published by Petite Marie Ltd
31 Underwood Rise
Royal Tunbridge Wells TN25RY
United Kingdom
www.petitemarieorganics.com

tel. +44 788 1830039

Printed in the United States of America

The views expressed in this work are solely those of the author and do not necessarily reflect the views of the publisher. The publisher hereby disclaims any responsibility for them.

The author hereby expressly disclaims any responsibility for any adverse effects that may result from use of advice and recommendations contained in this book.

ISBN-13: 978-1482364415
ISBN-10: 1482364417

To my little Maria, with love

# Praise for the Green Beauty Guide

**From Publishers Weekly:**

"In this thorough, practical guide, writer and registered nutrition specialist Gabriel (Clear Skin) recommends subjecting everyday cosmetics to the same scrutiny with which we subject our food.

Gabriel provides a list of dangerous ingredients to watch out for (and why), identifies the safest products on the market (free from 'synthetic dyes, fragrances, preservatives or detergents'), and takes readers step-by-step through cleansers, toners, facials, moisturizers, sunscreen, hair care and baby care.

Though aimed at women, Gabriel also covers products used by men and children, including shaving cream, soap, shampoo and powders."

"All hail to the lipstick revolution! Today, our world can't afford beauty without a conscience. Even our daily shopping habits that seem as mundane as our cosmetic and personal care product choices now have an enormous influence on our future. When shoppers read *The Green Beauty Guide* and put Julie Gabriel's insightful green beauty tips into practice, they are also being Green Patriot environmentalists, helping to build a safe and secure future for the world and for our children—not to mention improving their personal health and their appearance."

—David Steinman, founder of the Green Patriot movement,
author of *Safe Trip to Eden: Ten Steps to Save Planet Earth
from the Global Warming Meltdown.*

"Finally some sane and accurate advice about cosmetics and 'beauty products'! Julie Gabriel pulls no punches in this frank, honest, and totally unbiased masterpiece about the good, the bad, and the ugly sides of the cosmetic industry. Read this book because it could save your life."

— Dr. Zoltan P. Rona, MD, MSc, medical editor of
*Encyclopedia of Natural Healing.*

"I am often asked for a resource on cosmetics and ingredients. Julie's *The Green Beauty Guide* is an easy-to-read, informative introduction to many facets of the cosmetic world and how it connects to our well-being— from green to synthetic, do- it- yourself to super-expensive. If you are new to this world or even think you know 'green', step in and discover or rediscover this world and its underbelly."

—Suki Kramer, founder of *Suki Pure Skin Care*

"I would happily recommend *The Green Beauty Guide* to anyone wanting to learn more about their personal care products. It's easy to read, easy to understand, serves as an excellent quick reference guide, and will help move us all forward in our understanding of how and why we should re-examine what we're applying to our bodies."

—Terry Bly, founder of *FeelGood Style* (www.feelgoodstyle.com)

"Julie Gabriel has done a stellar job of creating an excellent resource that is powerful, thought-provoking, and incredibly bold. She challenges the system and encourages us to be diligent and informed about what we put on our bodies. Too often, as consumers, we complain to friends and ourselves but rarely do we take action. I think this book is an incredible show of force, and for the right reasons. Thank you, Julie, for this important tool. I cannot wait to give it to my family and friends."

—Anne Doulbeau, founder of *Inara*

"The definitive manual for any woman who wants to feel pampered and pretty while still maintaining an eco-friendly lifestyle. The book has an incredibly wide scope of information and deals with every aspect of our beauty regimen, including hair care, skin care, sun protection, cosmetics, fragrances, and even baby care."

—David Quilty, *The Good Human* (www.thegoodhuman.com)

"Once we read *The Green Beauty Guide*, we recycled all of our other organic beauty tomes—Julie is the definitive source and we never hit a beauty counter without her short list of product recommendations and ingredient red flags. Julie educates and inspires us to simply be more beautiful—we could spend hours making all of her fabulous DIY green beauty recipes. Read this book—your skin will thank you and so will your health!"

—Lisa Blau, Amanda Freeman, co-founders,
*Vital Juice (www.vitaljuice.com)*

# Contents

# Toners .................................................55

# Masks & Scrubs ..................................................................... 99

# Hair Care

## Bath Treatment

# Introduction

You are reading the much-asked-for sequel to my first book, *The Green Beauty Guide: Your Essential Resource to Organic and Natural Skincare, Hair Care, Makeup, and Fragrances* (HCI 2008). My first book provides quite a lot of theory: it tells you about artificial ingredients to avoid and why, which natural ingredients to look for, what makes them superior compared to synthetic counterparts, which organic products are truly green, and what makes them effective and enjoyable to use.

*Green Beauty Recipes* is all about practice. I am very proud and anxious to share with you my findings about how the organic beauty course of things really works, what makes natural cleansers so gentle, and how organic moisturizers actually moisturize—and what's even more exciting, how you can create them all by yourself, at very little expense, at home.

*The Green Beauty Guide* revealed some of the most dangerous sides of conventional, artificial, "junk food" beauty products. It told you what not to do. *Green Beauty Recipes* provides you with a blueprint on how to make the green leap and formulate your own cleansers, toners, moisturizers, and body products from scratch. You can use the finest organic raw materials, all-natural bases premixed by conscientious organic labs, or use kitchen staples directly from your cupboard. It's all up to you. No matter how much or how little you invest in your natural beauty ingredients, I am absolutely sure that the result will be gorgeous, green, and amazingly beneficial for your health and for our planet.

As a founder of Petite Marie Organics line of natural beauty products, formulated by me and loved by thousands of people worldwide, I have triple-tested each of the recipes. Many of the recipes presented in this book are currently used to make Petite Marie Organics cleansers, moisturizers, treatments, and baby products.

Green beauty is all about ingredients, not the media hype or sleek packaging. That's why using pure, raw, or minimally processed ingredients is very important. While it is tempting to me to give you a shopping list with some of the most expensive essential oils, peptides, and vitamins that could easily cost up to $1000 per ounce, I understand that this seemingly easy way will not work for all of us.

Some of the most effective recipes in this book cost only a few cents to make, and the ingredients are right there, in your kitchen cupboards, in your local grocery store, or maybe in your garden. My favorite facial oil is made from jojoba and tea tree oils; my favorite body polish is nothing but olive oil and fine sea salt with a sprinkle of mandarin essential oil for that uplifting fragrance; the most effective hair rinse and shine booster I have tried is simply apple cider vinegar. I make my own shampoos and baby bubble baths with Castile soap and a few affordable botanical ingredients.

Most of the recipes include a few optional ingredients, which add value and aid performance but may be more expensive. You can add them or skip them; the result will be just as good. Remember: you don't need to spend lots of money to look pampered, healthy, and gorgeous.

## What Makes these Recipes Different

If you choose organic, you do that because you care for your health as well as the wellbeing of our planet. However, with the abundance of organic frauds and gimmicks, it may be hard to tell the genuine organic or natural product from "greenwashed" wannabe products that put "organic" on the label without any true relation to the contents of their tubes and bottles. Today, a company can call its products "natural," even if they use 0.01% of natural ingredients in their product! Many of the recipes in the natural realm are full of artificial ingredients.

Here are ten things that make these recipes and the resulting products different from other natural recipes:

1. I want you to be able to create **environmentally friendly**, toxin-free beauty products that will make you heal-

thier and improve your wellbeing. There's not a single artificial or toxic ingredient suggested for use in these recipes.

2. Whenever possible, I recommend using **raw** or **minimally processed ingredients** that have been grown without synthetic fertilizers, pesticides, and stored without use of irradiation and synthetic preservatives.

3. Whenever possible, I recommend using ingredients that have not been **genetically modified**, especially when it comes to vegetable oils and soy-derived ingredients.

4. These recipes rarely contain ingredients from **animal sources**, such as gelatin, collagen, animal-based emulsifiers, and animal fats. Some of the exceptions include milk, yogurt, and beeswax.

5. At Petite Marie Organics, we do not support or commission testing of raw materials and finished products on **animals**. If possible, you should not purchase cosmetic ingredients from companies that do not have a clear policy against animal testing.

6. The recipes in this book contain absolutely **no** ingredients derived from **petroleum**.

7. I do not recommend using synthetic **preservatives**, penetration enhancers, talc, artificial dyes, or fragrances in any of these recipes.

8. Some recipes in this book call for the use of **alcohol**. I do not recommend using rubbing alcohol or denatured alcohol, because of the presence of carcinogenic toxins in these products. Instead, I suggest using distilled grain or grape spirit, such as vodka or grappa. Please make sure you have reached the legal drinking age for your country

before purchasing alcohol to use in recipes in this book.

9. Each recipe contains a **recommended shelf life**. To extend shelf life, you may refer to the segment on natural preservatives. Do not use the products that are past the expiration date, which you should clearly indicate on the packaging of the product, even if you plan to use them yourself.

10. These recipes have been **thoroughly tested**; some were approved by a dermatologist (doctor-vetted recipes are used in the production of Petite Marie Organics beauty products, yet I cannot offer you exact formulations for these products; there's such a thing as copyright.)

Your personal body chemistry is the only way to make sure that these recipes work for you. Your skin may react to certain ingredients, especially if you are taking prescription medications that may increase the sensitivity of your skin or if you have a family history of allergies. This is why patch test is the best way to make sure your homemade beauty preparation is compatible with your body chemistry.

## How to Do a Patch Test

How many times have you purchased a much-hyped product, only to discover that it caused almost blistering pain until you hurriedly rinsed it off, or that produced a cluster of pimples overnight? Just like it's nearly impossible to find a perfect beauty product that will faithfully serve you for many years, in winter and summer, in sickness and in health, it is even less possible to create a beauty product that would be perfectly tolerated by everyone. Due to the massive amount of chemical sensitizers bombarding us on a daily basis, we are more prone to allergies than ever. That's why I encourage you to perform a patch test each time you encounter a new ingredient or try a new formulation, especially if your skin is sensitive. Here is how to do the patch test properly:

1.  Choose an area in the crook of your elbow where your skin is more sensitive and sweat glands are abundant.

2.  Dilute the raw material with carrier oil or filtered water approximately in the same concentration as in the recipe. Do not apply essential oils or vitamins to your skin undiluted.

3.  Apply two drops of the mixture or raw ingredient with a cotton bud or a glass spatula. Cover with a band-aid and leave overnight.

4.  Next morning, carefully lift the bandage and look for any signs of an allergic reaction. Common symptoms include redness, warm feeling to the skin, rash, raised bumps, and itchiness.

If you are sensitive to an ingredient or a prepared product, please do not use it to avoid further reaction. You can always skip this ingredient in the recipe or substitute it for something similar. Many recipes suggest optional ingredients that you can use.

We are astonishingly ready to suffer in the name of beauty. As I was reading about the history of cosmetics, I was amused how happily women used poisons to achieve a "must-have" look of the day. In the eighteenth century, they smeared their faces with lead and mercury, lined their eyes with lead salts, scrubbed their teeth with pumice, and painted their lips with carmine. This willingness to suffer and even die in the name of beauty is nothing short of remarkable. It makes me wonder if there's a hidden flaw in human nature that makes discomfort, disease, and even death acceptable when it comes to looking attractive and desirable to the opposite sex.

But are women any different today? Today, to look and smell pretty, women are using poisons that are technologically advanced but equally toxic. Parabens, formaldehyde, toluene, quaterniums, aluminum, phthalates, ethoxylated dioxane-contaminated chemicals — all these beauty ingredients are just as toxic and deadly as lead, mercury, and ground marble.

Who knows, maybe fifty years from now our daughters and granddaughters will be equally amused at our willingness to spend untold amounts of money on synthetic cosmetics and paint our eyes and lips with makeup containing lead and synthetic pigments; fragrance our bodies with gender-bending phthalates; douse ourselves with lotions, shampoos, and shower gels containing parabens, formaldehyde, placenta, and vinyl.

This book is an introduction to making your own, personalized skin care products using all-natural ingredients suited precisely to the condition and concerns of your skin. You can make these products as natural and green as possible using certified organic, home-grown, or locally sourced ingredients.

For centuries, beauty products have been prepared from natural ingredients. Some of them, such as mercury or arsenic, were detrimental for your health; other, like rose oil, beeswax, and olive oil, have withstood the test of time and are successfully used in conventional and organic skincare today. But natural beauty products are so much more than olive oil or rose water. Today, thanks to the achievements of the organic trade, we have access to thousands of exciting elixirs, extracts, essential oils, natural vitamins, powdered plants, and distillates that offer tremendous benefits for our skin, hair, and overall wellbeing. To make our homemade creations more appealing and easier to use, we can add all-natural, plant–derived emulsifiers, humectants, and subtle penetration enhancers. To keep our creations fresh for longer, we can add a few drops of all-natural preservatives that protect from bacteria, fungi, and oxidation without toxic impact of conventional, synthetic preservatives, such as parabens.

Some products simply call to be made from scratch, while others require a bit of extra effort and time. As a working mom of a toddler daughter, I have very little time to concoct my moisturizers every week, so I use store-bought organic creams or the testers from my own organic line, Petite Marie Organics. But cleansers, toners, masks, scrubs, body oils, and hair treatments are incredibly easy to prepare, and if you make them at home, you are saving lots of money since you only pay for ingredients that normally cost a few pennies in a conventional skincare product. The rest pays for the packaging, storage, logistics, and multiple premiums that pay salaries to hordes of managers, sales people, and marketing professionals whose aim is to sell you another synthetic-smelling shampoo, not to make you healthier.

Another great thing about making your own skincare products is the possibility to adjust the product to your current beauty concerns. When you know which plant ingredients resolve your beauty concerns, you can twist and turn the recipes in this book to make sure they suit you precisely. You can make only an ounce of winter-specific facial oil to take you through the winter months, and for the summer time you can make another skin conditioner which will be better suited for hot weather and inevitable sun damage. This way, you get two perfectly natural products for the chunk of a price of a store-bought facial serum that will only deal with one or two skincare concerns. By making your own cleansers, toners, shampoos, and skin treatments, you can use only the ingredients that are helpful in this particular situation and skip the rest. You have complete control over what goes into the product (and what doesn't). Of course, you can make a product that will harm absolutely no animals, since you'll be testing them on yourself. If you use all-natural ingredients, there's little risk an animal suffered in their testing, too, because only synthetic cosmetic chemicals require thorough testing that kills rabbits and rats. Even if you rub olive oil onto a rat's skin, I doubt it will suffer much.

And if a recipe doesn't work for you, it's easy to wash it down the drain and make another version. When you become your own cosmetic chemist, the waste of time and money is minimal, while you become increasingly more mindful about your skincare and beauty in general.

## Important Disclaimer

The information published in this book is not intended to replace the advice of a medical care provider. Before making any decision affecting your personal health, please consult with your doctor, general practitioner, or a similar medical practitioner.

Please seek medical advice before using any herbal products, essential oils, or vitamins, especially if you are pregnant, breast-feeding, suffer from chemical sensitivity, take prescription medications, or suffer from a long-standing medical condition.

Please keep in mind that certain essential oils and herbal extracts may alter the performance of your medication. Please report any side effects to your medical practitioner. If an adverse reaction occurs, please discontinue using the cosmetic product immediately.

The statements in this book are provided for general information only. They are obtained from a variety of sources, including the research and personal experiences of the author. These statements have not been evaluated by the Food and Drug Administration (FDA). The products described in this book are not intended to diagnose, cure, treat, or prevent any disease.

*Recipes marked with an asterisk are used to formulate Petite Marie Organics skincare products (available at www.juliegabriel.com and www.petitemarieorganics.com, as well as select natural pharmacies). Please note that recipes in this book serve only as guidelines and are not exact formulations of Petite Marie Organics products.*

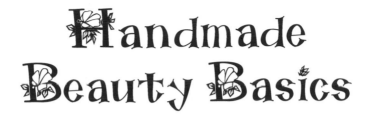

# Handmade Beauty Basics

In this chapter, we will look into the initial steps of handmade beauty creation. Whether you are a DIY beauty enthusiast or a salon professional looking to expand your product range, you will find useful tips and techniques on how to choose the ingredients, melt, blend, pour, store, and preserve your homemade green beauty products.

When I was starting my own beauty range, I was astonished at how little information was available on the sheer technicality of the process. You can find dozens of books on how to start your own fashion label, but there was zero on how to launch your own beauty line. My findings and revelations would have probably amused the industry veteran by their naiveté coupled with complete lack of respect to traditions and customs of the trade. I think it's all for better. If you don't know the rules of the game, you have no fear, too.

I learn new things every day. While I am grateful to technology for the progress in chemical-free sterilization and efficient storage, I may never leave it completely up to the machines to blend and homogenize my creams and lotions. Most Petite Marie Organics products are made by hand in small batches, and I'd love to keep it that way as long as possible.

To become a cosmetic kitchen chemist, all you need is a clean space, a storage rack or a cupboard (better yet, some clean space in your garage since it's naturally colder) for your ingredient stash, an electronic scale, a set of glass beakers, some Pyrex pans, and a stove. Helena Rubinstein and Estee Lauder started their brands right in their kitchens, so there's nothing wrong with following their example.

No matter where you plan to use these recipes — in your kitchen, garage, a home office, or an FDA-registered lab — cleanliness comes first when you deal with beauty products. Not only does your work space need to be sanitized and free from debris, but the equipment that you use must be sanitized at all times.

I do not encourage use of chlorine or triclosan-based disinfectants, including those containing chlorhexidine. Alcohol (ethanol) makes an excellent germ buster, but I do not recommend using rubbing (denatured) alcohol or any medical spirit, even though it is more traditional, because of its content of acetone and other harmful, volatile chemicals. You can buy a whole bottle of cheap vodka to cleanse your surfaces and equipment for much less than any brand-name sanitizer with tons of chemicals added for color and scent. To make the scent of the spirit less drinkable and therefore help you comply with the legislation, you can add at least three percent tea tree, eucalyptus, or peppermint essential oils to the blend. These oils will further improve the antibacterial action of your super-simple cleanser. For surface cleansing, vinegar is an excellent quick refresher.

I recommend using utensils and equipment made of stainless steel or medical glass. Wooden or rubber spoons or spatulas cannot be sanitized properly. Your utensils and equipment should be cleaned after and before every use. If you can afford it, an UV sanitizer is great, but a microwave oven is a convenient alternative. Microwaving kills all living matter, including germs. Do not put your steel spatulas in a microwave, though. Use alcohol to cleanse anything made of steel. To quickly cleanse the utensils you may wish to keep a spray bottle filled with vodka and a few drops of tea tree or eucalyptus essential oil. If you plan to decant the product into jars or bottles, sanitize them by microwaving or exposing to UV radiation and then add a quick wipe with alcohol just before pouring in the product.

Your working area must be well lit and ventilated. Ventilation is especially important if you plan to make more than an ounce of a product at a time. After dealing with various essential oils, especially when they are added to a heated product, you may feel a little woozy or even nauseous. If you feel unwell, quickly stop whatever you've been doing (even if it means that the cream would become stiff and require re-heating) and get a gasp of fresh air. If possible, lie down for a few minutes with windows open wide. Essential oils are no joke; they can provoke quite powerful reactions. For example, a certain blend of essential oils used in one of our bestselling products makes us all giggly and jittery for a few minutes, as we blend the product.

If you make beauty products just for your own use, you can skip the protective gear, but if you plan to sell your products, you must wear hairnets, gloves, and aprons or lab coats every time you handle supplies, equipment, products, or packaging.

Even though you will be using quite a lot of kitchen staples in your beauty preparations, ideally you should not consume food and drinks anywhere near your "organic beauty lab." If you work from your kitchen, this is not always possible. Please keep in mind that many essential oils are poisonous when taken internally, so you should keep them away from kitchen utensils, cutting boards, pots, and pans.

## How to Get Things Hot

To make creams, balms, salves, and soaps, you will need to heat and even boil a lot of natural waxes and butters. Some waxes and butters can be heated directly over low or medium heat, but this process may destroy some of the valuable phytochemicals and vitamins in the oils. Double-boiling is to direct boiling as steaming vegetables is to deep frying. Boiling water rarely becomes hotter than 212 degrees Fahrenheit (100 degrees Celsius). Not only does double-boiling preserve most of the important microelements in the ingredient, It also allows for more controlled mixing and blending as you heat the butter, wax, or oil.

A double boiler is simply a pot placed on top of another pot with boiling water in it, over a heat source. You can buy the pots already assembled or you can find two fitting pots in your kitchen. The pots should be cast iron, glass, or enameled steel. Never use aluminum or Teflon-coated pots and pans, as they will leach carcinogenic compounds in your skincare.

## Simple Double-Boiling Technique

1. Arrange two saucepans or a large saucepan and a Pyrex bowl (even a steel coffee pot would do), so that one fits loosely into another.

2. Fill the large pan with water so that the level of the water is approximately three inches below the rim of the smaller pan.

3. Place the wax or the butter into the smaller bowl.

4. As the water in the large bowl boils over medium heat, handle the large bowl with great care so that the water doesn't get into the melting ingredients.

5. Remove the double boiler from the heat source once the wax has turned into a liquid.

Another method of melting your waxes or butters is microwaving. While I do not recommend cooking your food in a microwave, it is a viable shortcut to quickly melt an ingredient for cosmetic use. Just make sure to microwave in a glass container, never in plastic, and to stand really far back from the device while it's working. Stir the liquid well to dissolve any hot spots.

Tip: to prevent grains from forming in your balms and butters, after heating and melting, cover your product and place it in the freezer for about ten to fifteen minutes.

## Water: Mineral, Flower, or Tap?

Water is the most abundant cosmetic ingredient. In an average moisturizer, water content reaches 80 percent! So if you care about the water you put inside your body, you should be just as careful about the water that will be soaked up by your skin.

Filtered tap water is perhaps the most economic and green solution. Jug filters like Brita will provide you with a reliable source of reasonably pure water to turn into toners, infusions, and moisturizers.

Mineral water can be tricky to work with. If you do want to add value to your products by using mineral water, make sure it is not too acidic because any variations in the pH can affect the viscosity of the finished product. Ideally, your mineral water should contain magnesium, silica, or calcium.

Flower waters and infusions are my favorite bases for cosmetic products. Flower waters, also known as hydrosols, are by-products of steam distillation of essential oils. Aloe water, however, is simply aloe juice squeezed from the inner parts of the stem. Fruit and vegetable juices, especially orange, grape, and tomato, make excellent bases for your homemade face, hair, and body treatment masks and baths.

## How to Steal the Soul of a Plant

There are many ways to reap the green goodness of your plant ingredients. You can buy the extracts ready-made, or you can play with your herbs and teas to make wonderfully fragrant and effective skin and hair preparations from scratch.

The most straightforward way to use skin-friendly plants is poultice. Poultices are effective for boils, acne eruptions, and even skin marks and scars. The process is super simple: chop the herb, crush the seeds, and then add a dash of boiling water to make a pulp. Place the pulp in a piece of cloth and apply to the affected area while hot. It should be replaced when the mixture cools down.

## Five Super Simple Poultices

- Potato wedges placed directly under eyes may help lighten eye circles.
- Cucumber slices placed on eye lids help relieve puffiness.
- Lemon slices may help lighten skin pigmentation.

- Sliced garlic helps shrink blemishes.
- A juicy apple may help revive the glow in tired skin.

An infusion is the most common way of preparing an herbal skin remedy. Infusions can be made with fresh or dried flowers, leaves, and soft stems. The simplest vessel to prepare an infusion is a china cup, a glass teapot, a coffee press, or a Pyrex bowl. Do not use a metal container! Place the required amount of the plant ingredient, fill the vessel with boiling filtered water, and put the lid on. Leave the mixture to steep for ten to fifteen minutes. Strain and use as directed in the recipe. If you need a stronger concentration of the active ingredients, increase the amount of herbs used, not the steeping period.

Plant bark, roots, and seeds are used to make a decoction. If you do want to extract active ingredients from hard plant matter, you will have to grind them with a pestle and mortar to break the cell walls, and then boil the coarse powder over medium heat for eight to ten minutes. As with infusions, strain and use as directed.

Infusions and decoctions can be used to make a compress. Soak a cloth in an infusion or a decoction, squeeze most of the liquid out and apply the hot cloth to the affected area. Compresses can be very little, covering your eyes or acne outbreaks; they can be very useful to treat sunburns and eczema on large areas of the skin.

Steams are similar to infusions. Steaming is very useful for skin problems like acne and dermatitis. To prepare a facial steam, add a handful of herbs, tinctures, or essential oils to boiling water, cover your head with a towel (optional), and carefully lean over the pan, exposing your skin troubles to healing vapors filled with volatile phytochemicals.

A tincture is the most challenging way to extract the active in-gredient from the plant. Technically speaking, tinctures are alcoholic extracts with ethanol percentage of up to 60 percent, but most often the concentration of ethanol rarely goes higher than 25 percent. I like working with tinctures because alcohol is chemically neutral and it offers an added bonus of being a mild preservative. However, for people who prefer not to deal with alcohol for medical, religious or moral reasons, non-alcoholic tinctures made with glycerin are a good alternative.

If you are lucky to have access to fresh skin-friendly herbs or simply want to flex your cosmetic chemist's muscle, here's how you can make your own tinctures for use in beauty products. Place the washed, roughly chopped herbs (you can mix and match them) into a medium-sized preserving jar and fill it with grain or grape spirit (vodka or grappa, ideally organic). Leave the jar to stand in a dark place for two to three weeks. Shake it occasionally to maximize the concentration of the active ingredients. When the tincture is ready, strain it and use to enhance your homemade beauty preparations.

You can use this technique to prepare infused oils for massage and body care (replace alcohol with any unscented plant oil) or glycerin extracts, also called glycerites.

Oil infusions can be prepared by hot or cold methods. For the hot method, fill a jar with fresh herb and cover with olive, grape seed, or sweet almond oil. Place the jar up to the neck in a saucepan of water and bring to a medium temperature. Simmer for up to three hours. Strain through filter paper or cloth into a brown glass bottle. For the cold method, place the jar with herbs and oil on a sunny windowsill. When the oil reaches the desired consistency, strain through cheesecloth or coffee filter (unbleached) and decant the oil into dark glass bottles.

## Working with Essential Oils

Essential oil is a volatile, strongly aromatic substance containing high concentrations of phytochemicals or "essence" of the plant. Essential oils have a long history of use in healing practices (aromatherapy), cosmetics, and fragrance making.

Essential oils are produced in one of three ways:

1. Water, or steam, distillation. In this method, heated steam passes through seeds, roots, bark, leaves, stems, or flowers, vaporizing the volatile compounds. The vapors then condense back to liquid, which is collected and used in cosmetic or therapeutic purposes. The water passed though the

plants is called hydrosol, hydrolat, herbal distillate or plant water essence, and makes an excellent skin toner or a water replacement in your cosmetic creations.

2.  Mechanical (cold) pressing of the peel of citrus fruits. Lemon, lime, and orange essential oils are produced by pressing the peel, which is a by-product of a fruit industry.

3.  Carbon dioxide (CO2) extraction is used to manufacture oils from most delicate plants. This way, the supercritical (liquid) gas acts as a solvent, which absorbs the volatile substances and phytochemicals from the plants. When the "essence" is collected, the pressure is reduced and the carbon dioxide reverts back to a gas, leaving no residue but a highly concentrated essential matter that can be used in skincare and fragrances. This matter is sometimes called an "absolute."

Essential oils have been used for cosmetic purposes for centuries, but most oils are too concentrated to be used straight, full-strength. Rose or jasmine absolutes are so overwhelmingly scented, one drop would be enough to turn a pint of vegetable oil into highly fragranced massage oil! That's why some of the most concentrated and fragranced essential oils and absolutes are turned into dilutes, that is, diluted with neutrally scented vegetable oils, such as sweet almond, jojoba, or apricot oils.

I recommend using only pure, all-natural essential oils in your green beauty creations. If the essential oil sold in a health food store or online contains a plant ingredient and an "aroma" or a "fragrance," you should not use it. Manipulated or semi-natural oils are not good for your skin.

Ideally, the ethical seller of essential oils should be able to provide you with a country of origin and a method of growing of plants from which the oil was extracted. Lavender essential oil from France is more expensive than lavender oil from England, and rose absolute from Bulgaria smells differently from rose absolute from Morocco. When given a choice, I prefer to buy oils from small traders or even directly from community farms and cooperatives working on fair trade principles. This way, you can get the freshest product at a reasonable price. If you buy from a large retailer, there's a chance that the oil may have been stored in a warehouse for many months, if not years, while small traders do not have the luxury of stocking very large quantities of products. On the other hand, large distributors and suppliers often carry their own product quality control and store their raw ingredients in appropriate conditions.

Your sense of smell is probably the most reliable and readily available tool to help you choose an authentic essential oil. It should not smell of alcohol or anything synthetic. If the smell is too harsh, then there's a chance the oil was "enriched" with artificial fragrances to make it more appealing. If a store has a sample vial for you to sniff at, note whether this vial smells a bit "off," and even stale. A natural essential oil will evaporate from being exposed to air many times a day. Semi-natural oil will smell bright and cheery, as if just opened. If a plant ingredient has undergone a drastic chemical transformation with synthetic chemicals, especially petrochemicals, it is not natural anymore.

Essential oils possess many healing qualities, working on your body and mind at the same time. Therefore, even if a recipe calls for use of certain essential oils, do not be forced to use them if you do not like their scent. By means of your volatile preferences, your body "chooses" the most beneficial substances for you to use at a particular moment. Trust your senses; if the oil smells offensive to you, do not use it, even if your recipe tells you so.

First and foremost, you should like the scent of your essential oils. Even if you think you cannot tolerate scents, most likely, you cannot tolerate chemical, synthetic fragrances. Almost everyone will eventually find an essential oil to fall in love with. For example, I buy some of my hydrosols from a small supplier in France. When I open their canister of cypress hydrosol, it envelopes me with such a true goodness of a sun-drenched, sea-kissed cypress grove at midday, I instantly feel like I'm on holiday. A high quality essential oil speaks directly to your subconscious — and that's the mystery behind all natural fragrances. After you get used to natural scents, synthetic fragrances in department stores will smell cheap and flat to you, like overpriced air fresheners.

Essential oils require little fuss with storage. A cold, clean place away from children and food is all you need. Ideally, your essential oil stash should have a lock on it because essential oils can be poisonous if ingested. Try to keep your oils in original cartons, if they were sold this way. Many essential oils are self-preserving and can be kept for up to two or three years. Most dilutes will go rancid after a year of storage, so try to use them up by this time.

Essential oils are power bombs of green skincare, and they must be used with great care. No matter which purpose you use them for, essential oils should never come in direct contact with your eyes or mucous membranes. Many essential oils are contraindicated for use in pregnancy and during breastfeeding. If in doubt, consult your health practitioner, and consider avoiding essential oils during these exciting periods of your life completely.

## Natural Emulsifiers

Emulsifiers are substances that are used to blend oils and water together to create a cream or a lotion by surrounding oil with tiny droplets and forming a protective layer so that the oil molecules cannot stick together. This way, an emulsion is formed. You can make it thicker by adding more emulsifier or thinner by using less emulsifier. Sometimes, you may even feel like adding an emulsifier to a facial toner so that you'll be able to add more essential oils without causing oil puddles at the surface! Egg yolk, honey, and mustard are common food emulsifiers.

An emulsifier is one ingredient that can make or break even the most natural product made with highest quality oils and mineral water. That's why if you plan to make creams, lotions, cleansers, and body creams, you need to make sure that your emulsifier is fail-safe and perfectly green.

Polysorbate and ceteareth (followed by a number) are frequently used in so-called organic beauty products, but these ingredients are not natural, and I do not recommend using them in your green beauty preparations. Polysorbate 20 is a polyoxyethylene derivative of sorbitan monolaurate, and ceteareth is a polyoxyethylene ether of cetyl alcohol or stearyl alcohol. You can use plain cetyl alcohol in your beauty products without any added petrochemical residue.

Emulsifying wax NF may sound natural but, in fact, it is anything but green and is certainly not natural. In fact, emulsifying wax is made of cetearyl alcohol, Polysorbate 60 (a petrochemical), PEG-150 stearate (another petrochemical), and Steareth-20 (yet another petrochemical). There's absolutely no reason to use this blend of synthetic chemicals in your natural beauty products!

Please note: if the ingredient name is followed by the initials NF, this means that it conforms to the specifications of the National Formulary, a manual containing a list of medicines that are approved for prescription throughout the country. So far, 156 countries have national or provincial essential medicines lists and 135 countries have national formulary manuals. NF often appears before "Emulsifying Wax," which may add importance but not naturalness to this ingredient.

Another emulsifier to avoid is borax (sodium borate.) Recent research shows it may be carcinogenic, and evidence-based research confirms that it is very irritating and allergenic. It also dries out delicate, mature skin, and is not recommended for use on children.

I have some bad news for vegetarians and vegans. Most emulsifiers used in cosmetic products are derived from animal fat. These days, legislation does not require listing the source of an emulsifier, just its chemical name, and these give no clue whether the emulsifier is derived from pig fat or not. So you can imagine how much pig fat goes into so-called natural and conventional beauty products! If you see the word "stearate" in your ingredient list, there's a good chance that the emulsifier was made from animal tallow, unless clearly labeled as vegetable.

And even if the emulsifier is plant-based, it cannot be certified organic, so to call a facial cream 100 percent organic is misleading, to say the least.

Making your own facial creams, lotions, and cream cleansers is the best way to avoid pig fat and petrochemicals in your beauty products. The best vegetable emulsifiers are derived from coconut or palm oils.

Glyceryl monostearate (glyceryl stearate) is a glycerol ester of stearic acid derived from shea or coconut butter. Make sure this emulsifier is marked as vegetarian before buying! Stearic acid can also be derived from animal tallow. If this is important to you, double-check with the manufacturer using contact information available online or on the packaging.

Cetyl alcohol is a popular natural emulsifier that is very easy to use. You simply melt it and combine with your oils and water. Or you can even skip oils to create an oil-free emulsion that will still be creamy and comfortable to use! Cetyl alcohol is a fatty alcohol derived from vegetable oils, such as palm oil and coconut oil. It is petroleum-free and is completely natural. In general, it is more suitable for thicker creams intended for use on dry, delicate, mature skin.

Sucrose laurate, a sugar ester of plant fatty acids, is my favorite plant-based emulsifier, and it is amazingly easy to use! Simply pour into the oil and add some water to get a wonderfully runny cream for an oilier or mixed complexion. And the best thing, it is approved for use in organic products by Soil Association, an organic certifying body in the United Kingdom.

Sodium stearoyl lactylate is made with lactic (milk) acid, stearic acid (make sure it's vegetable!), and then treated with sodium or calcium hydroxide. It must be used only in fat-in-water emulsions.

Cetearyl glucoside is made of corn-derived glucose and plant fatty alcohols. It is another failsafe emulsifier that is more suitable for products intended for use on mixed or oily complexions, and on the body. It will produce a lightweight, lotion-like texture with watery feel on the skin.

## Vegetable Oils in Your Beauty Products

Vegetable oils are the second most important group of ingredients in your green beauty products. If you shunned oils previously believing that they clog pores and make your skin oilier, this is because your skin has suffered from petrolatum and mineral oils so much, it reacts badly to all kinds of oils. Later on, I will introduce some of the most popular oils used in natural skincare.

Boiling is used to extract animal fats such as lard and tallow. I do not recommend using animal fats in green skincare.

The greenest method to extract a vegetable oil is cold pressing. During this procedure, seeds, nuts, and pulp are crushed and pressed. You can try and press a walnut in a garlic press at home: you will get a few drops of cold-pressed oil to use in your facial moisturizer. Cold pressing preserves all the vital benefits of plants in the oil. I only use cold pressed vegetable oils in Petite Marie Organics products.

Hot pressing is similar to cold pressing, but the plant matter is heated which helps it extract even more oil. However, most oils lose their phytochemicals and vitamins after heating, so hot pressed oils are good for mending squeaky doors, not in skincare.

When it comes to cosmetic use, plant oils can be soft and hard. In skin nutrition, saturated acids are heaviest, mono-unsaturated acids are medium-heavy and generally good for skin, and poly-unsaturated acids are thin, lightweight, and most beneficial.

The harder the oil, the less able it is to penetrate the skin, and more protective it is. Heavy, waxy oils form saturated acids in cocoa, mango, coconut, and shea butters, are used to nourish dry skin by preventing water loss from its surface. They also feed skin membranes with fatty acids and proteins.

Mono-unsaturated acids (also known as Omega 9) oils are also quite heavy but they can penetrate skin better than hard oils. Apricot, avocado, castor, macadamia, papaya, sesame, jojoba, and olive oils are used to lubricate and nourish dry to combination dry and normal skin, most often in face creams, body butters, body creams, and massage oils.

Thin and silky grape seed, sunflower, evening primrose, rosehip, pumpkin seed, walnut, and thistle oils form the poly-unsaturated acids group of oils that are most beneficial for delicate, mature, oily, and sensitive skin types. They are easily absorbed by the skin and leave no oily residue. Thin "dry" oils are non comedogenic (they do not clog pores.)

Beeswax is one of the very few non-plant ingredients that may occur in the recipes in this book. This hard and waxy substance is not absorbed by skin, but it creates a protective layer to protect from the elements. To make beeswax blend with your oils and water you need to heat it to the liquid point and then stir really well to make sure that it does not separate from the rest of the ingredients.

The heavier the oil, the longer it will keep fresh. Beeswax may keep fresh for up to ten years, although I do not recommend using it after five years of storage. Cocoa, coconut, and shea butters keep fresh for up to five years in cold, dark conditions. Most oils in mono-unsaturated group have a shelf life up to 4 years which can be reinforced with addition of wheatgerm oil or tocopherols, both natural antioxidants. Thin, delicate poly-unsaturated oils will only keep fresh for two years in dark and refrigerated conditions.

## Natural Preservatives

This is a very sensitive subject for me. At Petite Marie Organics we make products in small batches, and we even write the Best Before dates for each of the products, like for cheese or meat. If I add preservatives (or as they like to call them today, antioxidants), it is for the sake of our customers. I like to make sure that my products will keep fresh for a year or so in homes of our customers who often live in (or travel to) hot climates or store their skincare in warm humid bathrooms.

Preservatives ward off bacteria, fungi, microbes, halt enzyme activity, and slow down the oxidation of natural ingredients. The more preservatives that are loaded into the product, the longer the product remains potent, effective, and safe to use. You can avoid accumulation of toxins in your body by avoiding synthetic preservatives in favor of effective broad-spectrum preservatives which pose very little if any risk to your health.

In most conventional beauty products, preservatives may be used in a concentration of up to 5 percent of the formulation. And even so-called "organic" beauty brands may sneak through loopholes in organic legislation and use synthetic preservatives that they think are safe to use, sometimes despite current scientific evidence. Some artificial preservatives to avoid include:

Parabens
Triethanolamine
Phenoxyethanol
Ethylhexylglycerin
Denatured alcohol
DMDM Hydantoin
BHT (butylhydroxytoluene)
BHT (Butyl hydroxytoluene)
BHA (Butylated hydroxyanisole)
Benzyl alcohol
2-bromo-2-nitropropane-1,3-diol
Iodopropynyl butylcarbamate

Today, USDA Organics accepts only organic alcohol as a preservative in skincare products. I find this practice inappropriate. Products containing alcohol should not be used on babies because alcohol vapors may be seriously damaging to the fragile nervous system of babies and small children. To make alcohol an effective broad-range antioxidant and preservative, you need to use it in high concentrations up to 10 percent. This would make a cosmetic product too harsh for delicate, dry, and sensitive skin.

Disodium EDTA and tetrasodium EDTA are often used in "greenwashed" products. While these chemicals are used medicinally, there is no reason to use them in skincare. Both these preservatives are considered environmental pollutants, and in animal studies they appeared to be toxic to the DNA in living cells.

Another so-called natural preservative to avoid is sodium hydroxymethylglycinate. I know, it is hard to pronounce, and this is exactly the case: if you cannot pronounce it, don't put in on your skin. This preservative may be quite irritating, and its manufacturing process involves a lot of petrochemicals and other pollutants.

At the same time there are many broad-spectrum natural preservatives that will surely suit your beauty chemist's needs. They won't assure two or three years of storage in a warehouse, as parabens do, but they will extend the shelf life of your homemade beauty products for up to one year, especially if you store your products in clean, cool place and avoid exposing them to heat and humidity.

**Potassium sorbate** is derived from a reaction of sorbic acid with potassium hydroxide. It is a commonly used food preservative favored by winemakers. As a preservative, it inhibits molds and yeasts, kills microbes, and has no known adverse health effects. Potassium sorbate is non-irritating and non-sensitizing. Today, it is the most popular alternative to parabens. You must use 0.6 – 1.0 percent potassium sorbate in your green beauty formulations to extend the shelf life of your products by 12 months or even longer.

**Farnesol** is a natural chemical found in such essential oils as citronella, neroli, cyclamen, lemon grass, tuberose, rose, and tolu. It is a popular fragrance component with a sweet floral smell, and it is very popular in traditional perfumery. Only recently it was found that farnesol has antioxidant and DNA-preventive qualities. Interestingly enough, farnesol helps stabilize oil-based rich creams and massage oils and protects oils from going rancid.

**Aspen bark** (*Populus tremuloides*) extract is high in salicylic acid and may be useful as an additional preservative in your products for oily, congested, or unevenly pigmented skin. A powder that must be dissolved in water, aspen bark extract is good for emulsions, body mists, and toners. Due to the high content of salicylic acid, it is not suitable for people who are allergic to aspirin.

**Geogard** is the perfect preservative to use in serum and complex emulsions which can be challenging to keep stable. Containing naturally occurring gluconolactone and sodium benzoate (at very low concentration), Geogard can be added to the water phase without the risk of separation of the finished product. This preservative is approved for use in natural skincare (by Eco Cert) and is great to use in lotions, creams, bath and body cleansing gels, and hair care products, as long as they contain no ascorbic acid. The recommended dosage of this preservative is between 0.8 and 1.5 percent.

**Tinosan** (silver citrate and citric acid blend) is an easy-to-use broad spectrum preservative which uses an antibacterial action of positively-charged silver ions. Silver ions have broad-spectrum antimicrobial activity and are effective against unwanted skin bacteria, yeast, molds, and pathogenic microorganisms. Silver citrate is not the same as colloidal silver and is not toxic because it does not accumulate in our tissues. "It is well established that only silver in its ionic or complexed forms is antimicrobially active, while the elemental silver, even in the so-called "nanocrystalline" state is not. Silver-containing compounds are attractive because of the fact that in the range of the applicable concentrations, silver ions do not exhibit toxicity and carcinogenic activities," Canadian biochemists wrote in 2008 (Djokic, 2008). Tinosan is especially useful in water-based toners, shampoos, and deodorants. You should use it in a concentration of 0.3 - 0.6 percent.

If you are making products for your own use or to sell in a spa setting, you may be comfortable using silver citrate, but if you plan to sell online, please note that many countries and eBay.com do not allow silver compounds in skincare products, based on the tarnished reputation of colloidal silver.

All of these preservatives will extend the shelf life of your products by months if not years. If you aren't looking to make your homemade green beauty creations by batches, you may wish to consider even simpler options.

**Vitamin E** (tocopherol) is a very useful antioxidant that can prolong shelf life of your products for up to 12 months if added in a concentration of 2%. It works synergistically with vitamins C (ascorbic acid, ascorbyl palmitate) and vitamin A (beta-carotene or retinol), both added at concentrations of 0.5 - 0.8 percent. These vitamins act as antioxidants and are very useful in anti-aging, anti-acne formulations or in homemade sun products but to be truly effective you may consider using another broad-spectrum preservative in addition to vitamins.

**Rosemary** (Rosmarinus officinalis) leaf extract and essential oil are good sources of antioxidant terpenes. They help protect the product from "premature aging," that is, from oxidation. You may use 0.15 – 0.5 percent rosemary extract or essential oil in your formulations.

**Grapefruit** (Citrus sinensis) seed extract is often sold under the name "citricidal" which is a blend of grapefruit seed extract and glycerin. It is a fairly foolproof antioxidant that may help extend the shelf life of your products by six months or more. You can add this compound generously, but keep the concentration under 1.5 percent.

Many essential oils such as açaí, caraway, cinnamon, clove, coleus, cumin, eucalyptus, lavender, lemon, lemongrass, niaouli, oregano, rose, rosemary, sage, sandalwood, tea tree, and thyme have antioxidant action and may serve as a natural alternative to preservatives. The chemical benzanthracene found in lemon and lime oils have potent microbial properties. If you use some of these oils in your formulation, you may need to worry less about added preservatives. You may even concoct your personal effective blend of antioxidant essential oils to use in your own beauty products.

Many beauty products do not require preservatives at all. Water-free face and body balms, face, bath and body oils, oil-based body scrubs, body and hair butters, liquid soap (water-free), bath salts, body powders, and soaps can be stored for up to 12 months without any preservatives. And of course, you can carefully watch the way you handle your beauty products. Store your natural beauty products in cool, clean places, promptly close the containers, and if possible, use spatulas or Q-tips as applicators instead of fingertips.

## Green Beauty Packaging

Nearly all organic and natural skincare brands continue using plastic containers despite the fact that plastic requires more natural resources to recycle than glass, and not all types of plastic containers can be recycled. Many types of plastic can leach plasticizers such as phthalates and vinyl to the products. Still, plastic containers have their benefits. They are lightweight which is good for travel and it keeps shipping costs low. If you choose to use plastic, look for polypropylene (PP) and high-density polyethylene

(HDPE). Polyethylene terephthalate (PET) bottles are more ubi-quitous but they can leach phthalates into the product, especially if there are acidic ingredients in the formulation. Some companies carry double-walled jars which have polypropylene inner contain-er and a pretty glass-looking polyethylene terephtalate (PET) outer shell. These containers are great for prolonged storage of products but they may not be easily available in smaller quantities for a home beauty enthusiast.

While many proponents of plastic claim that plastic is better because it doesn't break and therefore is safer than glass in the bathroom, I have not had a single broken cosmetic or baby feeding bottle in my bathroom with stone floors in three years of use. Glass does not leach chemicals into the products, and it is easily recyclable. For formulations with high content of essential oils I recommend using dark-tinted glass such as cobalt blue, amber, purple, or green. Lotion bottles with pumps are great for liquid serums and lotions, especially sun protection products. I have listed some good sources of glass bottles and jars in the Appendix A.

Glass jars from kitchenware stores such as Mason jars have certain rustic appeal, but I found them too awkward to use in the bathroom although they look great as containers for body scrubs and bath salts. They are useful for soy candles and potpourri, too.

No matter which material you choose for your jar, keep in mind that cleanliness is vital. Sterilize the jars and bottles in a microwave or with a UV sterilizer for salon equipment if your homemade preparations do not contain any preservatives or additives. But since you most likely have great pride in your cosmetic achievements, you would want to use them often and generously, so you would finish the batch long before it has a chance of becoming rancid.

The greenest way to obtain containers for your homemade beauty products is to reuse glass and plastic containers that you already own. Take a good look at your existing skincare stash; chances are, some of your serums, creams, and masks are past their prime or have simply expired. Wash them thoroughly and sanitize with rubbing alcohol or grain spirit. For my custom-made products I use white glass containers from Crème De La Mer products and dark glass Estee Lauder serum vials even though I no longer use conventional skincare products. To prolong the shelf life, use a tiny spoon or spatula to retrieve the product from the container, instead of scooping it out with your fingers, and store the large batch in the refrigerator, decanting only the amount you need for week's use in a small mini-sized container.

## Storage of Natural Beauty Products

Ingredients and finished products should be stored and handled carefully. Everything must be clearly labeled with the name of the product and the lot number. All containers should be tightly closed at all times. All containers should not be stored directly on the floor. You should make certain that you are storing your ingredients and products in an area that does not expose them to excessive heat or cold, sunlight, or moisture. A product improperly stored will cause it to age prematurely, oxidize, and go rancid or moldy too quickly.

Each recipe in this book has a suggestion regarding the shelf life. As a rule, all masks containing fresh fruit, vegetables, eggs, dairy, and honey should be used within one day from preparation. Masks with clays especially if they contain antioxidant essential oils and plant extracts can be stored for up to a week in the refrigerator. Foaming cleansers can be stored for up to six months depending on the amount of essential oils and vitamins used in the formulation. Oil-based facial serums can be stored for up to six months in cool dry conditions and water-containing moisturizers can be stored for up to three months unless you add natural preservatives to extend shelf life. Bath salts can be stored for up to a year in a tightly closed container. Body oils and oil-based scrubs can be stored for up to a year, too, but ideally your must use them within six months from blending to ensure that your botanical ingredients are fresh and potent.

## Green Beauty Labels

If you want to give away or sell your homemade beauty creations, a legible waterproof label is a must. You can find good quality white or clear polypropylene or polyester labels at stationery retailers and online. Steer clear of vinyl labels that emit formaldehyde when you print them on a laser printer. Most labels come with ready-made templates for the ease of design in your favorite graphic design program. However, if you simply want to share your homemade beauty goodies with family or friends, feel free to add Kraft paper tags with cute handwritten messages hanging on some lovely string or a silk ribbon. No one expects your homemade beauty to look as sleek and polished like department store skincare bottles!

Labels also work to warn others that the product is actually skincare, not food or a toy. A few years ago, I sent my friend (a new mommy) a large bag of LUSH skincare products that contained bath bombs, salts, and scrubs looking like candy canes, muffins, yogurts, and cookies. I soon found out that my gift was not accepted well. Apparently, when my friend has put the bag with fresh cosmetics into the refrigerator, her toddler son ate or at least tried every product that looked like a candy or a muffin. The little explorer didn't get poisoned. He didn't eat a lot of foaming bath salts because of a bitter taste. But I have learned my lesson. Food and beauty don't mix; even if I make beauty products completely edible, with food ingredients, they should be clearly labeled as skincare immediately after preparation.

## Where to Buy Ingredients

All ingredients used in the recipes in this book are easily available from grocery stores, supermarkets, drug stores, health food stores, and online retailers. You will find lots of useful resources in Appendix A to this book. Many ingredients can also be found right in your kitchen cabinets or a pantry. Organic olive oil from the grocery store is more affordable than similar olive oil from a cosmetic ingredients retailer. Ground almonds, oatmeal, ground rice, semolina flour, and corn flour are widely available in super-markets and groceries. Organic grape and grain spirits can be added in small quantities to deodorants and astringents.

The greenest way to source the ingredients is to grow them yourself. Melissa, mint, lavender, chamomile, calendula, and many other herbs and flowers can be easily grown in your garden or on the window sill. You can dry the leaves, stalks, petals, and whole flowers for use in bath preparations, soaps, and masks, and you can prepare infusions to use in cleansers, toners, and treatments. With a little experience, you can also prepare tinctures that have long shelf life thanks to the presence of alcohol.

## What is Green Beauty?

Over the years, we have been conditioned to believe that only liquids packed in vacuum, triple-walled containers with a posh logo on the label are able to properly cleanse, nourish, and revital-ize our skin. This whole book tries to prove three important things: that beauty is indeed food for our skin; that beauty product doesn't have to cost a lot to make a difference in your skin and hair condition; and that going green, at least when it comes to skin and hair care, is surprisingly cheap.

Skincare is food for our skin. The way you take care of your skin tells me a lot about the way you eat. If someone mindlessly picks the most attractive, heavily advertised box from the glitzy department store counter, this person would most likely prefer to eat in a posh restaurant without much care of what really goes into his or her steak or a tiramisu. Such people don't have a clue whether their food was made from organic, non-GMO, or at least free-range, local ingredients, as long as it tastes good and looks impressive on a plate.

If someone's diet consists of soda, chips, chocolate bars, and French fries as the only source of their "five a day" recommended intake of vegetables, they are likely to slap any fast-food beauty product from the drugstore isle, as long as it smells good and promises eternal youth at a reasonable price.

If you, like me, scrutinize every ingredient on the cereal box, then you will scrutinize the ingredients in your beauty product with same suspicion and care. If you cook your meals from scratch, recycle, buy local in season and in bulk, something tells me you are likely to pop the leftover yogurt on your face or whip up a simple body scrub from olive oil and sea salt. This book will teach you at least 200 more ways to prepare gorgeous beauty products from your kitchen staples and some other easily available natural ingredients.

## Green Beauty on the Run

When I do my weekly grocery shopping, I make sure to pick up some foods that can be used in homemade cosmetics. Not only they make great additions to your weekly menu, they are also packed with skin- and hair-friendly ingredients. Here is a list of food products (and two drugstore staples) one-step green beauty recipes that you can make instantly from the ingredients in your fridge and kitchen cupboards.

**Avocado**: a ready-made, preservative-free remedy for dry skin, split hair ends, and rough cuticles.

**Baking soda**: makes a great face and body scrub when mixed with olive or any other oil; can also be used as grainy exfoliating filler for your more intricate masks and scrubs; when added to bath water, softens the skin.

**Chamomile tea** can be used as a toner, hair rinse for blonde hair, and a general purpose calming skin and hair mist.

**Cocoa**: great face mask and hair rinse for dark hair.

**Coffee**: the contents of your coffee filter can be used as a body scrub; very strong brewed (cool) coffee is a great hair rinse for dark hair.

**Corn flour**: soothing, tightening, and mildly exfoliating agent for masks and scrubs.

**Eggs**: can be massaged into the hair as a nourishing conditioner; egg whites are a traditional face lifting remedy.

**Epsom salt**: great for relaxing bath that would soothe itching skin and revive the muscles.

**Green tea**: a great all-purpose skin toner, face mask and scrub filler, eye soother, and a baby skin rinse if your little one suffers from eczema.

**Honey**: an antibacterial ingredient, a soothing face mask, and very useful cure for dandruff - just add some honey to your shampoo.

**Lemons**: juice makes a gorgeous skin whitening and hair lightening treatment; rind can be used to scent the bath water; oil squeezed from the rind works magic on acne blemishes.

**Milk of magnesia**: very effective mask for acne, sun burns, and eczema.

**Mayonnaise**: gorgeous moisturizer for face, body, and especially feet.

**Milk**: use it to wipe your face after cleansing for mildly exfoliating effect; add to bath water to soften the skin; rinse your hair for added volume and to combat dryness.

**Oranges**: cut them in half and add to your bath water along with olive oil.

**Vegetable oils**: should be your number one beauty ingredient. Vegetable oils can be added to the face cream, as a massage oil, bath oil, or body/face scrubs. Great skin-friendly oils to explore include grape seed, rice bran, hemp, castor seed, jojoba, and sesame oils.

**Sea salt**: works great as a face and body exfoliating agent, especially useful for instant manicures. Look for very fine sea salt which will not damage your skin.

**Sugar**: fine brown sugar can be used in face and body scrubs.

**Oat bran** and **oatmeal**: make them into scrubs, face masks, bath pouches.

**Tomatoes**: revive tired skin and hair to help it look shiny and smooth.

**Yogurt**: works really well as an exfoliating face mask and to combat dry, itchy scalp.

# 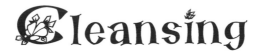Cleansing

Our facial skin is perhaps the most vulnerable skin area on our bodies. Our faces are constantly exposed to harmful elements. We can cover the skin on our bodies with clothes, we can cover our hand with gloves and mittens and our hair with hats and scarves, but our faces are out there, facing the sun, pollution at all times.

Cleansing is a very important step of any beauty routine. If you don't cleanse your skin thoroughly, none of your next steps, such as toning, exfoliating, moisturizing won't have much effect. Regularly and thoroughly cleansed skin will retain its beauty for many years to come. Without proper cleansing, your moisturizers and topical treatments will not be able to deliver their active ingredients and may even make your skin look worse by clogging up already blocked pores.

When we cleanse, we do not simply remove "dirt" which accumulates minute by minute, all day long. In the morning, we cleanse the pores from the accumulation of stale sebum and dried sweat with all the toxins flushed to the skin surface during the night. In the evening, we rinse off the makeup, sunscreen residue, particles of dust and soot, dried sweat, dead skin cells and bacteria, and many other ghastly things that cling to our epidermis and may eventually seep into the dermis and further into the bloodstream. That's why the ideal cleansing routine should gently exfoliate, massage, and nourish. In the perfect world, you shouldn't need any additional beauty products after you have properly cleansed your skin.

There are three basic types of cleansers: a foaming gel, a milky lotion, and a cleansing oil. Each of these types can be transformed into an exfoliating cleanser by adding a pinch of jojoba beads, fine sugar, fine sea salt, semolina flour, fine oatmeal, almond meal, or ground rice. Even green tea from packets can become a mild brightening exfoliating agent. Take a look around your kitchen and become a creative beauty cook.

When you make your own skincare, you can afford the luxury of having one cleanser for the winter and one for the summer, a foaming cleanser for heavy makeup days, a milky cleanser for no-makeup days, a powder cleanser for a bit of exfoliating, a cleansing oil to use when your skin feels a little dry and flaky; and a mixture of all of the above when you are feeling a little bit like experimenting and inventing something new and exciting.

## Natural Cleansers in Detail

In essence, a natural foaming cleanser consists of three major groups of ingredients. First of all, it is water or a water replacement such as herbal infusion or a hydrosol. Second, the cleanser must contain a cleansing agent to dissolve the grime and carry it down the drain. And third, a good cleanser may contain softening, antibacterial, or exfoliating ingredients.

Here are some of the most popular foaming bases for your homemade cleansers.

**Castille** and liquid **Marseille** soaps are perhaps the greenest option. Castille soap is made with olive oil treated with potassium salts, while Marseille soap is traditionally made by mixing sea water from the Mediterranean Sea, olive oil, and potassium salts. You can buy liquid olive soaps online or in good health food stores. They usually blend well with oils, exfoliating granules, and plant extracts. Most of them do not disperse granules well, so they tend to fall down to the bottom of the bottle. If this happens, shake your exfoliating cleansers before use.

**Cocamidopropyl betaine** (cocobetaine) is derived from coconut via somewhat not so green manufacturing process involving petrochemicals. Still, it's fairly natural but exactly organic. This anionic surfactant is gentle and easy to use, and it can be a blessing for a beginner beauty chemist. Cocobetaine blends well with other surfactants if you decide to use them to increase foaming in your bath products or shampoos. By itself, it foams lavishly and cleanses well without drying out your skin. You should use no more than 6% cocobetaine in your formulations.

**Decyl glucoside** is made from plant fatty alcohols and glucose.

When purchased from a reputable retailer, it should not contain any harmful impurities. Decyl glucoside is very mild and you only need to use a dash to make good foam. You can combine it with cocobetaine for stable foaming of your cleansers, body washes, and shampoos. Caprylyl/capryl glucoside is similar in composition but may be used alone due to its mildness and good soft foam.

As a rule, avoid surfactants with words laureth or similar -eth in the name. You don't need any ethoxylated compounds in your homemade green skincare! Similarly, avoid surfactants with diethanolamides, lauryl sulfates, laureth sulfates, parabens, or formaldehyde in your beauty formulations.

# Basic Foaming Cleanser Formula

*This formula is suitable for facial, hair, and body cleansers, if you like soft, smooth, stable foam. Feel free to modify it to adjust to your needs by adding exfoliating agents, essential oils, plant extracts, and vitamins.*

## Ingredients

### Phase A
50 percent filtered water, hydrosol, or plant infusion
2 percent glycerin

### Phase B
40 percent surfactant A (liquid olive soap)
6 percent surfactant B (cocobetaine and/or decyl glucoside)

### Phase C
0.6 percent vitamins A, C, E (or other preservatives of your choice)
1 percent essential oils

## Method

Phase A: Combine and stir/homogenize until completely dissolved. Castile soap may form transparent globules when diluted with water. Stir well until your mixture is uniform.

Phase B: Combine and mix well. Add to Phase A and stir thoroughly.

Phase C: Combine with rest of the ingredients with good mixing.

This product will produce lots of foam if whisked briskly. To avoid this, stir slowly in a circular motion. Allow to settle before packaging.

It is very easy to adjust the foaming cleanser to your skin's needs by adding more oils, vitamins, or exfoliating agents, such as jojoba granules, rice beads, or clay. If you decide to add clay to your foaming cleanser, make sure to blend thoroughly, using a stick blender, but the result will be worth it.

**Cleansing oil** is best made with lightweight oil, such as sunflower or jojoba, and may also contain a natural emulsifier, such as sucrose laurate, so that it will form an emulsion when mixed with water. This will help rinse the cleansing oil. You may add antibacterial or antioxidant essential oils to the blend.

**Cleansing lotion** (milk) is essentially a very thin lotion that lifts off the grime and makeup and forms an emulsion, which will be easily rinsed or wiped off. Cleansing lotions are best used for dry skin and around the eyes, especially if you need to remove waterproof makeup (in this case, cleansing oil is also very useful).

**Rhassoul clay** (mud) should be mentioned as a cleanser in its own right. It is a unique, very absorbent clay containing water trapped inside clay particles that deliver silica, magnesium, potassium, and calcium. Thanks to the high mineral presence, rhassoul clay is great for problem skin or dandruff-prone scalps. To use as a shampoo, take 1 tablespoon, depending on your hair length. For facial cleansing, ½ teaspoon is quite enough. It rinses clear and even foams to some degree. Rhassoul mud doesn't blend too well with surfactants, but it is an excellent ingredient to use on its own.

After years of negative press, soap is regaining its glory as a facial cleanser. Today, natural soaps are made without pore-clogging animal tallow and skin-drying harsh lye. You can make your soap from scratch using some of the fabulous online recipes and books on soap making.

# Nourishing Skin Cleansing Oil

*Wheat germ oil is an excellent natural preservative, thanks to the high content of vitamin E. When added to the cleansing oil, it extends its shelf life to one year. This simple cleanser can even be used to remove makeup around the eyes, and castor oil helps nourish eyelashes and encourage their growth.*

## Ingredients

> 1 oz castor oil
> ½ oz grape seed oil
> 1 tablespoon wheat germ oil
> 5 drops geranium essential oil

## Method

> Pour the oils into a dark glass bottle using a funnel, close the lid, and shake well to mix.

## Application

> Apply with cotton wool or clean fingertips. Gently wipe in a circle from the inner corner of the eyelid towards the hair line. To wipe off the long-wearing makeup, saturate a cotton wool and rub gently, then rinse off with warm water and follow with a foaming cleanser, if desired.

## Storage

> This oil can be stored up to eighteen months in a tightly closed, dark-glass container.

# Purifying Cleansing Oil*

*Conventional cleansing oils often contain petrochemicals and synthetic emulsifiers that allow easy rinsing. If you use thin, "dry" oil, such as jojoba, thistle, or hemp, it will still rinse easily without leaving your skin feeling dry and taut.*

## Ingredients

2 oz jojoba oil
1 oz thistle or hemp oil
15 drops tea tree essential oil
10 drops lemon balm essential oil
5 drops chamomile essential oil (optional)

## Method

Pour the oils into a dark-glass bottle using a funnel, close the lid, and shake well to mix.

## Application

To use, warm a few drops between your palms and massage your face, avoiding eye area. Remove with warm washcloth or rinse off with water, then follow with a foaming cleanser, if desired.

## Storage

This oil can be stored up to twelve months in a tightly closed, dark-glass container. Replace the cap promptly after use.

# Delicate Skin Soap

*Good-quality Castile soap is not too foamy and turns milky when rinsed off. However mild by nature, it can be a bit too drying for super-sensitive, delicate skin. You can soften Castile soap by adding vegetable oils and herbal glycerites to it.*

## Ingredients

2 oz Castile soap
¼ teaspoon oats glycerite
¼ teaspoon vitamin E
1 tablespoon aloe vera juice

(OPTIONAL)
10 drops chamomile essential oil
5 drops rose absolute essential oil
5 drops melissa (lemon balm) essential oil

## Method

Combine all ingredients in a container of your choice and shake well.

## Application

Rub a quarter-size amount between your palms to make foam; massage into your face to remove makeup and cleanse your skin.

## Storage

Up to three months in a closed container.

# Carrot Cake Cleansing Cream

*This gentle cleanser is suitable for dry, sensitive skin, possibly with eczema. Coconut oil leaves the skin soft and feeling slightly cool, which is great for eczema sufferers. Rosemary and carrot seed oils act as natural preservatives.*

## Ingredients

1 oz orange water
½ oz coconut oil
⅓ oz beeswax
⅓ oz vegetable glycerin
½ oz semolina or almond meal
10 drops rosemary leaf extract
5 drops carrot seed extract
3 drops vitamin E

## Method

Heat the orange water in a double boiler until very hot. Double-boil coconut and olive oils along with grated beeswax until liquid. Slowly and carefully pour the heated orange water into the hot oils, beating with a fork until fluffy. Blend in the grains of your choice. Add the glycerin. Continue beating until soft and creamy. Add the essential oils and vitamin E only when the mixture cools down and reaches the temperature of your skin.

## Application

Warm a few drops between your palms and massage your face, avoiding eye area. Remove with warm washcloth or rinse off with water, then follow with a foaming cleanser, if desired.

## Storage

Six months in a cool, clean place, away from light.

# Aromatherapeutic Facial Cleansing Gel

*Frankincense, juniper berry, honey, and fenugreek are just some of the ancient anti-aging remedies used to condition and heal the skin. This gel is non-foaming and is suitable for very gentle, sensitive skin that cannot tolerate foaming cleansers.*

## Ingredients

3 oz water
½ teaspoon xanthan gum
2 tablespoons white clay (kaolin) or Fuller's Earth
10 drops frankincense essential oil
10 drops juniper essential oil
2 teaspoons honey (optional)

## Method

Heat the water until warm, then carefully sprinkle xanthan gum on its surface while whisking briskly. While the water is still warm, add the clay and whisk or use a stick blender to prepare a runny custard-like substance. Add essential oils and honey and blend more. Transfer to a bottle.

## Application

Every morning and evening massage a quarter-size amount into your face and neck, then rinse well.

## Storage

Store up to three months in a closed container. Replace the cap promptly after each use.

# Sunshine and Lollipops Liquid Facial Soap

*Buttermilk powder acts as a wonderful source of fatty acids, while plain olive liquid soap serves as a great neutral base for essential oils. The scent is adorable. You can use it to cleanse your face, body, and hair. If you are sensitive to the members of the ragweed family, please skip chamomile essential oil.*

## Ingredients

   3 oz olive, Castile, or Marseille liquid soap
   1 oz buttermilk or baby formula
   1 tablespoon glycerin
   2 tablespoons honey
   5 drops mandarin essential oil
   3 drops neroli essential oil
   2 drops rose essential oil
   1 drop chamomile essential oil

## Method

   Combine the ingredients in a pump bottle and shake or stir well until the milk disperses thoroughly. You may wish to heat the mixture slightly to achieve a more homogenous mixture.

## Application

   Massage two pumps into your wet face and rinse with tepid water.

## Storage

   Store up to six months in a cool, clean place, away from sources of heat.

# Good Morning Cleansing Rub

*This gentle scrub exfoliates and soothes dry, taut skin. Soy milk is a great vegan alternative to dry dairy milk and it is less comedogenic.*

## Ingredients

1 cup traditional oatmeal
1 teaspoon olive or sweet almond oil
2 tablespoons powdered soy milk or cow's milk.
Optional:
If you want to use this rub on your body, you may add
1 tablespoon organic brown sugar.

## Methods

Combine the ingredients in a bowl and stir well to make a nice runny paste.

## Application

Rub your face with one to two tablespoonfuls of the mixture; leave on as a mask to dry. Meanwhile, eat the leftovers, because this rub cannot be stored.

## Storage

This rub can be stored in a refrigerator for only one day, so prepare just enough to use in the morning and in the evening.

# Oats, Almonds, and Olive Face Cleanser

*Extra virgin olive oil blended with apple cider vinegar make much more than a salad dressing. They do wonders for adult impure skin, too! Avoid using plain white wine or malt vinegars, which tend to be chemically processed. You can also make your own herbal vinegar for your cosmetic and culinary use by soaking fresh herbs, such as mint, rosemary, sage, or thyme, in apple cider vinegar for two to three weeks. Herbal vinegars can be used in this recipe.*

## Ingredients

1 tablespoon fine oatmeal or almond meal
1 tablespoon wheat bran
1 tablespoon honey
½ cup vinegar
½ cup olive or grape seed oil

## Method

Combine all ingredients in a bowl and stir well to make a light, creamy fluid. Transfer into a bottle with a pump dispenser.

## Application

Every morning or evening, apply one pump (one teaspoon) of the mixture onto your wet face and massage well. Let the cleanser sit on your skin for a minute before rinsing off.

## Storage

You may store this blend for up to two weeks in a closed container in a refrigerator or in a cool, clean place.

# Coconut and Neroli Cleansing Balm

*This is a soothing makeup remover that deeply nourishes dry skin. Natural plant butters work to dissolve the daily grime and even waterproof makeup with ease, while essential oils and vitamin E nourish and revitalize tired complexions.*

## Ingredients

2 oz cocoa butter
2 oz extra virgin coconut oil
10 drops neroli essential oil
10 drops vitamin E oil (tocopherol)
8 drops lavender essential oil
5 drops vanilla extract or essence

## Method

Melt the butter and oils in a double boiler. Allow them to cool to body temperature before adding essential oils and vitamin E. Transfer to a glass jar and allow to cool down to room temperature.

## Application

Every morning or evening, use a hazelnut-sized amount to lightly massage into your face. Avoid getting the balm into your eyes. Rinse with a face cloth and warm water.

## Storage

Store up to three months; please keep the container tightly closed.

# White Clay Skin Lightening Cleanser

*Montmorillonite clay, also known as Fuller's Earth, has mild skin-whitening properties, while lemon juice and chamomile are traditional facial brighteners.*

## Ingredients

Juice of ½ lemon
2 oz natural olive oil soap
1 oz montmorillonite or white clay
10 drops chamomile essential oil

## Method

Squeeze the juice from the lemon and strain. Add to the soap and whisk gently to avoid excessive bubbles forming. Gently fold in the clay and stir well. Use a stick blender if needed. Add the essential oil and stir more.

## Application

Every morning or evening, use a hazelnut-sized amount to lightly massage into your face. Avoid getting the cleanser into your eyes. Rinse off with a face cloth and warm water.

## Storage

Store up to three months; please keep the container tightly closed between uses.

# Juicy Fruit Foaming Cleanser

*Apple juice is rich in natural acids that gently slough off dead skin cells while feeding your skin with enzymes, vitamins, and antioxidants. You can combine Castile soap with grapefruit, grape, and orange juice or create your own fruit cocktail combination. Just make sure to add no more than one part juice per four parts of soap.*

## Ingredients

4 tablespoons apple juice
1 oz natural olive oil soap
1 oz green clay (illite)
OPTIONAL: 10 drops chamomile, mandarin, lemon, and/or carrot seed oil. If using all four, make sure you do not exceed 20 drops essential oil for 1 ounce of Castile soap.

## Method

Combine juice and soap and stir gently to avoid excessive bubbles forming. Gently fold in the clay and stir well. Use a stick blender if needed, but keep it below the mixture level otherwise you'll get tons of bubbles! Add the essential oil and stir more.

## Application

Every morning or evening, use a hazelnut-sized amount to lightly massage into your face. Avoid getting the cleanser into your eyes. Rinse off with a face cloth and warm water.

## Storage

Store up to one month in a refrigerator or in a cool, clean place. Please keep the container tightly closed.

Green Beauty Recipes

# Peach and Lime Exfoliating Facial Soap

*Alpha hydroxy acids in peaches and limes, as well as other citruses, help soften wrinkles, sun spots, age spots, and blemishes, and can even unclog pores. If you want to seriously lighten your complexion, double the amount of limes in this recipe. You can buy ready-made soap flakes or finely grate any organic or all-natural soap you fancy.*

## Ingredients

> 1 medium peach
> 1 lime
> 1 cup soap flakes
> 1 tablespoon fine sea salt

## Method

Peel the peach and remove the stone. Finely chop it or make a puree with a food processor. Squeeze the juice from the lime and add to the peach puree. Stir well. Fold in the soap flakes and the sea salt. Stir well to achieve a homogenous mass. Transfer to a glass jar.

## Application

Every morning or evening, use a hazelnut-sized amount to lightly massage into your face. Avoid getting the cleanser into your eyes. Rinse off with a face cloth and warm water.

## Storage

Store up to one month in a refrigerator. Please keep the container tightly closed between uses.

# Celery and Hamamelis Eye Wash

*In ancient Egypt, a common eye wash was prepared with celery juice and hemp oil. This eye wash can be used to remove makeup and also to prepare soothing compresses for sore, red eyes and to reduce puffiness.*

## Ingredients

2 celery stalks or 2 tablespoons celery juice
1 green tea bag
2 cups witch hazel (Hamamelis)
1 tablespoon glycerin

## Method

Puree two celery stalks in a food processor and strain the juice from the pulp. Alternatively, extract the juice using a juicer. Place the teabag in a glass beaker. Heat witch hazel until hot and pour it on top of the teabag. Let the tea infuse for two to three minutes, then remove the teabag and discard it. Add celery juice and glycerin. Stir well and transfer to a container.

## Application

To wipe your eyes, saturate a cotton wool disc and gently cleanse the eye lid and the eye area. Avoid pulling your skin. To make a soothing eye mask, saturate a gauze pad and apply to the eye area for ten to fifteen minutes.

## Storage

Keep refrigerated for up to ten days. Discard immediately if the mixture becomes cloudy.

# Rose and Oats Cleansing Cream

*Any natural liquid soap combines beautifully with a Basic Cream 1 (see page 74) to make a nourishing yet thoroughly cleansing facial wash for dry, delicate skin. I prefer to add rose otto and oats glycerite to this blend; you may come up with more creative ideas. This cleanser is best used in winter time.*

## Ingredients

- ½ cup Basic Cream 1
  1 cup natural liquid soap, such as Castile soap
  5 drops rose otto essential oil or
  4 tablespoons rose hydrosol
  10 drops oats glycerite or an oats tincture

## Method

Prepare the cream using the recipe in Chapter 3. Combine with the soap while the cream is still runny and hot. Stir well to form a creamy substance. It may harden as the cream cools down. If using rose hydrosol, add it while the cream is still hot and stir well. If using rose otto, add when the cream is pleasantly warm to the touch. Add oats glycerite and stir well. Transfer to a glass or plastic jar.

## Application

Every morning or evening, use a hazelnut-sized amount to lightly massage into your face. Rinse off with a face cloth and warm water.

## Storage

Refrigerate up to one month; keep the container tightly closed.

# Quick Green Cleanser Ideas

Organic **full-fat milk** is the ultimate quickie cleanser. Just pour some milk on a cotton wool ball and wipe off the eye makeup and refresh the skin. There is no need to wash the milk off. Top it off with your regular moisturizer or leave it as it is and enjoy a mild exfoliation, as milk sours it gives your skin a natural glow.

**Baby formula** and **almond meal**, mixed in equal proportions, make a great natural scrub.

Many **baby cereals** work as wonderfully gentle cleansers. Just mash the leftovers from your baby's breakfast with a few drops of olive or sweet almond oil and spread over your face, massage a little, and rinse off.

**Yogurt**, which contains mildly exfoliating lactic acid, makes an excellent antibacterial cleanser.

**Oatmeal** by itself makes a wonderfully gentle buffing cleanser. You can use it plain with a few tablespoons of hot water, but make sure not to scald your face! Hot water is needed just to soften the oatmeal.

To remove waterproof or mineral makeup, saturate cotton wool with **virgin olive oil** or **grape seed oil** and gently wipe off the mascara and eye shadows.

When your skin rebels over lack of sleep, abundance of stress, or the junk food diet, try milk of magnesia. Use a plain variety, without added sugar or flavors. Apply **milk of magnesia** with a cotton ball after you have removed makeup with facial oil or soap. Leave the liquid on for a few minutes and rinse off.

When it comes to non-abrasive scrubs, nothing comes close to juicy, ripe **papaya**. Papaya skin contains an enzyme called papain that helps to remove dead skin cells and loosen skin impurities. With regular use, papain helps fade post-acne marks and blotchiness caused by sun damage. After cleansing your face, peel a ripe papaya and rub the inner side of its skin directly all over your face while avoiding the eye area. Leave on for five to ten minutes and rinse with tepid water.

# 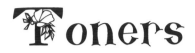oners

Toners are used after the cleansing and before applying the moisturizer. They act as astringents and may help reduce the look of pores and wrinkles. They may also soothe and purify the skin by removing last traces of cleansers and makeup removers. You absolutely need a toner if you are using cleansing oils or cleansing lotions.

Toners are very helpful in achieving your skincare goals. Dry skin can receive additional soothing and nourishment from plant infusions and vitamins. Oily skin can be purified and rebalanced after cleansing. Sensitive or fragile skin can be soothed and calmed with the use of some of the most gentle plant juices and mineral water. And anyone can benefit from a facial mist made of mineral water blended with birch juice or rose water on a hot summer day or when leaving a gym.

Herbal infusions are simple and yet surprisingly effective facial toners. You can use them on dry and sensitive skin, and if you have oily skin or acne breakouts, you may add a little apple cider vinegar. Infusions are very easy to make — same as you'd make a cup of tea. If your skin is in trouble, I recommend using an infusion twice daily after cleansing and also preparing a suitable mask in the base of the infusion of your choice.

Most toners can be blended easily right in the container. To store your toners, I recommend glass or polypropylene containers with a small spout or a spray top. This way, you can spray the toner directly on your skin or on the cotton wool disc, thus eliminating its contact with air. It helps prolong the toner's shelf life and maintain its effectiveness.

# Rejuvenating Face Toner

*Apple cider vinegar helps restore glow to flaky, impure skin. It also helps maintain skin's natural acid mantle, which protects from skin infections. Honey is another time-tested skin purifier, while glycerin soothes and moisturizes. Due to the acidic nature of this preparation, I recommend wearing sunscreen daily to prevent uneven pigmentation.*

## Ingredients

1 cup filtered water or chamomile tea
½ cup apple cider vinegar
1 tablespoon honey
½ teaspoon vitamin C powder
1 teaspoon glycerin

## Method

Add vinegar, honey, and vitamin C powder to the tea. Stir well to disperse vitamin C. Add glycerin and stir or shake well.

## Application

Every night, wipe your skin with a cotton ball soaked in this toner.

## Storage

Store up to three months in a cool, dark place.

# Double Apple Toner

*Use this toner to exfoliate and purify oily, blemished skin. Apple supplies anti-bacterial pectin and a host of vitamins and minerals. One apple a day (the Green Beauty way!) will surely keep the derma-tologist away!*

## Ingredients

3 oz apple juice
1 tablespoon honey
3 tablespoons apple cider vinegar
5 drops tea tree essential oil

## Method

Core (don't peel) the apple and coarsely chop it. Combine all the ingredients in the blender. Blend all ingredients using a stick blender. Strain through coffee filter paper and pour the toner into a container.

## Application

Shake well before use. Smooth over the face, avoiding eye area. Rinse off with tepid or cool water.

## Storage

Store up to one month in a clean, cool place.

# Soothing Water for Sensitive Skin

*This multi-tasking formula can be used in masks and as a toner for easily irritated skin and flaky scalp. Neroli water is generally well tolerated, even by people who are sensitive to citrus oils. Rose helps soothe inflammation in the skin, while carrot juice and green tea help diminish puffiness and redness.*

## Ingredients

1 cup water
1 green tea bag
½ cup neroli water
½ cup rose water
3 tablespoons carrot juice

## Method

Place the tea bag into a beaker cup. Boil the water and pour it on top of the tea bag. Cover the cup with a saucer to prevent phytochemicals from evaporating. Meanwhile, measure all waters and juice and combine them in a bottle. Remove the tea bag from the beaker and discard it. Strain green tea through a coffee filter and add it to the rest of the ingredients. Shake or stir well to blend.

## Application

Use twice daily or as often as needed. This formula can also be used to make a hair rinse.

## Storage

Store up to two weeks in a refrigerator.

# Age Rewind Skin Toner

*Alpha lipoic acid (ALA) is a well-studied antioxidant that protects your skin from elements, both when taken internally as a supplement and when applied topically in skincare products. It is important to use very little of this ingredient, as it can cause stinging when used in abundance. If you buy ALA as a supplement in capsules, keep in mind that capsules often contain lots of fillers, such as cellulose and anticaking agents, which may affect the look of your product. You can purchase pure alpha lipoic acid from many online retailers that cater to natural beauty enthusiasts.*

## Ingredients

> 1 cup witch hazel
> 1 cup filtered tap water
> 1 tablespoon glycerin
> ½ teaspoon Echinacea tincture
> 2 mg alpha lipoic acid

## Method

> Combine all ingredients in a polypropylene or glass bottle (not PET!) and shake well until ALA crystals dissolve.

## Application

> Apply twice daily after cleansing. Avoid the eye area.

## Storage

> Store up to twelve months in a clean, dark place.

# Milk and Olive Facial Toner

*Ancient Greeks used honey to moisturize their faces and olive oil to protect their skin from sun and other drying elements. This toner best suits dry, sensitive skin.*

## Ingredients

2 cups water
½ cup milk
3 tablespoons olive oil
1 tablespoon glycerin

## Method

Combine all ingredients in a container, replace the cup, and shake well.

## Ingredients

Use twice daily after cleansing or as often as needed. Shake well before use.

## Storage

Store up to one week in a refrigerator.

# Herbal Toner for Oily Skin

*This strong toner is very useful to remove the last traces of long-lasting makeup and concealers, to lift up pore blockages (comedones) in skin pores, and to restore the skin's protective acid mantle.*

## Ingredients

1 cup witch hazel
1 cup strong black tea
3 tablespoons apple cider vinegar
1 tablespoon grain alcohol

## Method

Combine all ingredients in a glass bottle and shake well.

## Application

Apply this toner with cotton wool in upward strokes, avoiding eye area. Let the toner evaporate and penetrate, leaving your skin dry, before applying a moisturizer or a treatment serum of your choice.

## Storage

Store up to twelve months in a closed container.

# Almond Milk Toner

*When your skin feels dry at one spot and oily at another, you don't need to use two or three products at the same time. Soothe and nourish your skin and allow it to rest while it heals.*

## Ingredients

½ cup rose water
½ cup almond milk
1 tablespoon glycerin

## Method

Mix all ingredients together in a bottle and shake well. Shake well before each application.

## Application

Gently apply to the whole face, including the eye area. Do not rinse.

## Storage

Store up to two weeks in a refrigerator.

# Skin Detox Toner

*Witch hazel is a time-tested astringent and antioxidant. It helps soothe skin inflammation and reduce visible pore size. Lemon and lime juices help brighten and lighten the skin, but please keep them away from the eye area.*

## Ingredients

1 cup water
2 chamomile tea bags
½ cup witch hazel
2 tablespoons lemon or lime juice
½ teaspoon cornstarch
5 drops lavender essential oil
5 drops rosemary essential oil

## Method

Boil the water. Place teabags in a cup and pour the water on top. Let the tea infuse for five to seven minutes, then remove tea bags and discard them. When the tea cools down, combine it with witch hazel, citrus juice, and cornstarch. Stir well. Add the essential oils and stir more. Transfer to a bottle.

## Application

Apply to clean, dry skin, avoiding eye area. Do not rinse.

## Storage

Store up to one month in a refrigerator or in a cool, clean place.

# Skin Brightening Toner with Sake

*Sake is a Japanese rice wine containing whitening enzymes that gently exfoliate and brighten your complexion. Green tea is a strong antioxidant, while rosemary sprigs help preserve the mixture and soften the smell of sake.*

## Ingredients

Make sure you have reached the legal drinking age in your country before purchasing ingredients for this recipe.

3 oz green tea prepared in filtered or mineral water
2 oz sake
3 fresh rosemary sprigs

## Method

Prepare green tea by steeping one packet of tea in a small cup covered by a saucer. Place rosemary into a bottle. Add green tea and sake mixture. Shake well to mix. Leave in a cool, dark place for 24 hours for rosemary to infuse the blend.

## Application

Apply to clean, dry skin, avoiding eye area. Do not rinse. Follow with a sunscreen if using in the morning.

## Storage

Store up to one month in a cool, clean place.

# Layer Cake Clay Toner

*This is a double-phase toner that has to be shaken, not stirred, before use. It helps soak up excess oil and prevent acne breakouts. It is not recommended for dry or sensitive skin because it can leave delicate complexions feeling dry and tight.*

## Ingredients

2 cups water
1 cup chamomile hydrosol
½ ounce witch hazel
3 tablespoons white clay
2 drops cedar wood essential oil
1 drop frankincense essential oil

## Method

Combine water and hydrosol, and then carefully add clay. Shake well. Add essential oils and shake more.

## Application

Shake before use and apply to the T-zone with a cotton wool disc.

## Storage

Store up to twelve months in a glass container.

# Ten One-Step Toner Ideas

**Orange juice** is a great toner for oily, dull-looking, congested skin. You can use orange juice straight from the carton on a cotton wool disc.

All **vegetable juices** are great as toners, too. Try **celery, potato**, or **cabbage juice** to revive lackluster skin. **Pomegranate, orange, grapefruit,** and **grape juice** make excellent toners that are rich in vitamin C, antioxidants, and astringent phytochemicals. Freshly pressed juices are best, but juices from concentrates also make great toners. You can blend them with **green tea** or add a few drops of **grain alcohol** for astringency.

Any **tea**, including **white, green, rooibos, mate,** and **black tea** makes a great toner that feeds your skin with powerful antioxidants.

**Milk** is a great toner, too. Wipe your face with full-fat milk to reveal nourished, visibly clearer skin in less than a week.

**Milk of magnesia** is a great toner for skin that suffers from an onset of adult acne. Leave the milk of magnesia overnight to visibly diminish blemishes.

**Witch hazel** is a traditional toner for oily, impure skin. You can add witch hazel to virtually any toner (except those for sensitive skin) to extend shelf life of your toner and make it more effective.

**Sea water** (often sold as a nasal spray in large bottles) is even more beneficial for your skin than mineral water. It is especially good for lifting and toning sagging, mature skin.

# Moisturizers

In this chapter, you will learn how to create the most essential item in your skincare arsenal—a moisturizer. This chapter will show how moisturizers are created and what the key elements in a cream, a lotion, or a balm are. You can refer to this chapter as we go ahead and learn the recipes for sun products, baby care, and body care products.

All skin types benefit from moisturizing, even the oilier skin types. In oily skin, the production of sebum has been compromised by excessively drying skin treatments, so that you need to approach this skin type with utmost care and moisturize it with lightweight, oil-based, non-comedogenic serums and naturally oil-free moisturizers based on natural humectants, such as soy lecithin, maltodextrin, various glucosides, plant-derived squalane, and hyaluronic acid. Whenever a natural emulsifier is present, make sure it is derived from a plant source, as many emulsifiers either come from petrochemicals or animal fat.

Why do we need a moisturizer? First of all, it helps prevent water loss by locking some of the water inside our skin cells with oils and waxes. Moisturizers also replenish the water already lost by excessive evaporation and taxing lifestyles by attracting water from the outside environment using humectants, some being as simple as sugar and plant glycerin, and some being more complex, such as olive-derived squalane, seaweed-derived vegetarian hyaluronic acid, and birch-derived xylitol. Moisturizers also supply our skin with essential fatty acids to maintain healthy, resilient skin cells, and antioxidants to prevent DNA damage in skin by free radicals.

Plant oils are the simplest and perhaps most effective moisturizers know to cosmetic science. In fact, most commercially available moisturizers are made of tiny amounts of plant oils mixed with abundant amounts of water, emulsifiers, penetration enhancers, and preservatives. All of these ingredients are less expensive than plant oils, so it's no wonder that a regular "synthetic" moisturizer would contain four percent plant oil (which does the moisturizing job), seventy percent water, with the rest being chemical junk that holds together a teaspoon of oil and a cupful of water, preservatives, and perfumes.

That's why, whenever my skin is in trouble — too little or too much sunshine, PMS, cold spells, dry spells — I reach for one of the undiluted oils in my cosmetic lab. Just a few drops of a pure oil could do the job overnight. If I travel and have no access to rare oils, such as chia, açaí, papaya, or raspberry seed oil, I use olive and castor seed oil, both commonly available in pharmacies, groceries, and supermarkets.

This is not to say that rare oils, such as moringa, açaí, blueberry seed, or argan are just as good as plain olive oil. Oils from smaller plants tend to be more concentrated in rare essential fatty acids, antioxidants, and vitamins. Certain oils are helpful for serious skin conditions and often help make a dramatic difference without the use of prescription drugs.

Many less-popular oils, such as jojoba, hemp, or thistle oils, are indispensable for oilier skins because they are so fine and almost dry to the touch; they disappear instantly in the skin, leaving no oily residue. In fact, the skin feels a little matte and dry, which of course is a blessing for oilier complexions. Still, you can rest assured your skin is getting lots and lots of vitamins and healing essential fatty acids.

## How to Apply a Moisturizer

After cleansing your skin, splash your skin with a toner or pat your face dry. Apply your cream or a lotion in gentle upward strokes without pulling your skin. Spread it evenly, using gentle massaging strokes. Always moisturize your neck using just as much product as on your face. Your neck shows signs of aging just as quickly as your eye area. But if you can use some drastic measures to diminish wrinkles around your eyes, you can do absolutely nothing to take years off your neck area. There are too many important blood vessels lying close to the skin surface and the thyroid gland is located in such close proximity. No one would safely inject anti-aging shots into the neck area for this reason. That's why you should protect your neck from aging starting at age 30 by applying a rich antioxidant cream at night and a sun-protecting cream during the day.

All natural moisturizers are emulsions created by blending water, vegetable oil, and an emulsifier. Other ingredients, such as vitamins, plant extracts, and essential oils, are added to the emulsion for their healing, soothing, or purifying properties. You can make an oil-free moisturizer by blending water, a gel-making agent such as xanthan gum or cellulose, along with some lightweight emulsifier, adding botanicals and vitamins to suit your skin condition.

Creating a good emulsion requires precise measurement. In this chapter you will also learn what to do if things go wrong and your emulsion doesn't look or feel right. As you gain more experience, you will be able to adjust the recipes to your liking and create even better formulations. In my own practice, not a single batch of creams or lotions is similar to another, no matter how precisely we follow the recipes. That's perhaps the difference between handmade and machine-made skincare. Every single jar of natural handmade cream is unique and precious to us.

And speaking of measurements, please note that recipes in this section will yield approximately 3.3 fl oz (100 ml) finished product. If you need to make a bigger batch, please feel free to multiply the recipe. You can vary the outcome of the recipe by adding more or less water or active ingredients.

## Water in Moisturizers

You can use filtered tap water or mineral water, as long as it contains very little mineral salts that can interfere with the way the emulsifier works. I recommend using tap water filtered via a regular jug filter and then further purified using a super absorbent microcarbon mineral shungite (part of Petite Marie Organic Beauty Water Kit, available at www.juliegabriel.com). This mineral will absorb organic compounds (including pesticides), metals, bacteria, and harmful microorganisms, and produce gallons of pure, scentless, crystal clear water that is richer in minerals than distilled water.

# Vegetable Oils and Butters

For centuries, people used vegetable oils, waxes, and butters to moisturize their skin and hair, protect it from elements, and create colorful cosmetics. Unlike mineral oils and other petrochemicals, vegetable oils, especially cold-pressed ones, enrich the skin and hair with essential fatty acids and do not interfere with skin metabolism. All vegetable oils make wonderful bases for home-made moisturizers, cleansers, and balms, but some of these oils are more suited for your unique complexion than others.

As a rule of thumb, waxes and fatty oils are not easily absorbed by skin and are more protective and nourishing. Semi-fatty oils are both nourishing and lightweight, which makes them versatile and easy to use. Dry oils are lightweight and easily absorbed by skin without any residue at all. They are most suitable for oily skin and hair care.

Here are the ten most popular oils used in skincare, along with recommendations for their skin type compatibility. You can read more about oils and their health properties in my book *Green Beauty Ingredients: 850 Most Effective Oils, Herbs, Minerals, and Vitamins to Use in your Natural and Organic Skincare, Hair Care, Makeup, and Fragrances.*

**Apricot kernel** (*Prunus armeniaca*) oil is a semi-fatty, un-scented, and non-comedogenic oil that is suitable for all skin types, including mature and sensitive. It is easily absorbed by the skin without greasy residue. This oil can be used in moisturizers, cleansers for dry skin, and massage oils.

**Avocado** (*Persea gratissima*) oil is a rich, semi-fatty oil with a mild nutty aroma. It is rich in beta-carotene and vitamins B, D, and E. It is useful for dry, mature skin and body care.

**Castor** (*Ricinus communis*) oil is a very fatty, heavy oil that is not easily absorbed by skin. It is very useful in lip care, massage oils, and face balms and ointments. Castor oil is surprisingly effective against acne, but may be comedogenic.

**Coconut** (*Cocos nucifera*) butter is a lovely fragranced, solid oil that melts on contact with skin. It is fatty oil that may be comedogenic in some people. It is not easily absorbed by skin, which makes it an excellent addition to cleansing balms, hair cleansers, and body care products.

**Jojoba** (*Simmondsia chinensis*) is a plant wax that is fatty, protective, and yet non-comedogenic. In moisturizers it traps water inside the skin without clogging pores, which is great for people who are prone to acne. This oil helps create self-preserving balms and moisturizers for all skin types.

**Olive** (*Olea europeana*) oil is a semi-fatty rich oil that softens and protects skin and hair. Olive oil is rich in antioxidant phytochemicals and essential fatty acids. It is beneficial for combination/dry skin and body massage oils.

**Sesame** (*Sesamum indicum*) is a mildly scented, semi-fatty oil that is very beneficial for all skin types, including very sensitive. It can be used for baby massage, as a hair oil, and in moisturizers for all skin types.

**Shea butter** (*Butyrospermum parkii*) is a fatty oil with time-tested nourishing, healing, and protective properties. It is beneficial for skin irritations, in sun products, and during flare-ups of eczema, acne, and dermatitis. Refined shea butter is scentless, unrefined butter has a distinctive, nutty aroma.

**Sunflower** (*Heliantus annuus*) is a semi-fatty oil that is great for skin prone to inflammation thanks to the high content of anti-inflammatory essential fatty acids. This oil is easily absorbed by skin and is not comedogenic. Sunflower oil can be used on combination/oily, oily, and sensitive skin, including for babies.

**Thistle** (safflower, *Carthamus tinctorius*) is a thin, dry oil that is absorbed rapidly without any greasy after feel. It is unscented and well tolerated by sensitive skin. It can be blended with jojoba and sunflower oils for use on oily, inflamed skin and flaky scalp conditions.

## Natural Moisture Boosters

To make a moisturizer truly effective, you need more than a good-quality vegetable oil or a wax that will trap the water in the skin by preventing its evaporation. There are several amazing substances that can attract moisture from outside and help lock and retain water inside the epidermis for a prolonged period. These ingredients are called humectants.

**Glycerin** (glycerol) is the easiest to use humectant with a good scientific track record. It is non-irritating and well tolerated by sensitive and acne-prone skin. Clear and odorless, it mixes well with all ingredients and helps prolong shelf life of your homemade beauty products. Pure, vegetable-derived glycerol may be used for soothing and lubrication of psoriasis, bites, cuts, rashes, and calluses. Glycerin blends well with water and can be used in thin emulsions, as well as cleansers, toners, and masks. The recommended concentration is three to five percent.

It is very important to buy glycerin from a reputable provider. Since the early 1990s, a toxic component, diethylene glycol, was discovered in some synthetic, i.e., petroleum-derived, glycerin-containing products. You should only use vegetable-derived glycerin made by a reputable manufacturer in your beauty products. Ideally, your glycerin must be organic so that its origins may be traced. Please refer to my hand-picked list of suppliers of organic ingredients in Appendix A.

Please also note that I cannot be held responsible for any changes in product selection, prices, or ingredient lists offered at suggested retailers and suppliers.

**Sorbitol** (glucitol) is a naturally occurring sugar alcohol that is commonly used as a laxative and a sugar substitute. Sorbitol is chemically synthesized from starch and glucose. Like glycerin, it helps skin retain moisture and remain supple and soft, but unlike glycerin, which leaves skin silky and slippery, sorbitol creates a velvety, shine-free feel to the skin. You can use this humectant in moisturizers, masks, and hair products. You can buy sorbitol syrup at most pharmacies and many online stores. The recommended concentration is two to four percent.

**Panthenol** (pro-vitamin B5) is a great humectant with soothing and healing capabilities. It works by strengthening the surface of the skin or hair, making it less able to expel water. It also binds water in deeper layers of the skin and may even help speed up skin regeneration, which makes this ingredient indispensable for skin suffering from acne, sunburns, and skin infections. The recommended concentration is two to four percent.

**Hyaluronic acid** (*sodium hyaluronoate*) is a new humectant that is gaining popularity. Like glycerin, it is clear, unscented, and easy to use. It is very effective in retaining moisture inside the skin, which helps smooth wrinkles and plump the skin. If you are vegan, look for hyaluronic acid that is not derived from animal sources, such as rooster combs. Instead, look for vegetarian hyaluronic acid derived from seaweed. The recommended concentration is one to four percent.

There are many so-called "naturally derived" humectants that I do not recommend using in your natural beauty products. These include carbamide (urea), caprylyl glycol, ethylhexylglycerin (often comes in a preservative blend,) various PEGs (polyethylene glycols), and propylene glycol.

## Making Basic Natural Moisturizers

Each time I make a cream, I am fascinated by the alchemical aura surrounding this process. Three liquids are turned into fragrant custard in a matter of minutes! Making your own moisturizers is a fun, creative, and incredibly personal process, during which you can make your own formulas from scratch by following a few simple rules. Here's the process of making any emulsion, be it a thick cream for dry skin or a thin lotion for body care. Please refer to these recipes and use these methods when you make your own moisturizers, masks, and scrubs; sun care products; baby care products; body care; and hair care products.

The recipes will produce approximately 3.3 oz (100ml) of product. There are two basic methods for making a cream: one for use with natural emulsifiers and one for use with beeswax.

# Basic Cream 1

## Equipment

Two double boilers
One stainless steel whisk or one hand-held stick blender
One measuring glass
Two measuring spoons or electronic scales
Kitchen thermometer

## Ingredients

### Fat Stage

0.3 oz (10ml) vegetable oil
4g emulsifier (cetyl alcohol)

### Water Stage

2 oz (60 ml) water, aloe vera juice, or hydrosol
2 ml/g glycerin
0.5 ml preservative of your choice (optional)

### Value Stage

25 drops / 1 ml essential oil (single or a blend)
2 ml/g vitamin E oil
30 drops plant glycerol of your choice

## Method

Heat the Fat Stage ingredients in a double boiler until all ingredients are melted and the temperature has reached 176°F (80°C).

In your second double boiler, heat the water to the same temperature (176°F / 80°C), gradually adding glycerin and a preservative, if using.

Turn off the heat under both double boilers. Pour the melted Fat Stage ingredients into the Water Stage. Pour slowly in a thin stream and continuously whisk the mixture clockwise for five minutes. You can also use a stick blender but please be careful to avoid splattering the boiling hot liquid on yourself.

Allow the mixture to cool naturally without using fans or placing it in a fridge. Stir with a stainless steel spoon or a spatula until the mixture reaches desirable consistency without clumps.

After the mixture has cooled to 104°F / 40°C (pleasantly warm to the touch), add all Value Stage ingredients except the essential oils.

When the mixture has cooled to 86°F / 30°C, add essential oils and blend thoroughly.

Spoon or pour the mixture in a jar and label it, noting the time of preparation.

If you want to make a lotion for cleansing, face care, or body care, you can dilute the Basic Moisturizer with an appropriate hydrosol or an herbal infusion.

# Basic Cream 2 (with Beeswax)

## Equipment

One double boiler
One stainless steel whisk or one hand-held stick blender
One measuring glass
A measuring spoon or electronic scales

## Ingredients

### Wax Stage

A bar or unrefined or sun-bleached beeswax

### Fat Stage

2 oz (60 ml) vegetable oil / a blend of oils of your choice

### Water Stage

1 oz (30 ml) water, hydrosol, or herbal infusion
2 ml/g glycerin
0.5 ml preservative of your choice (optional)

### Value Stage

25 drops / 1 ml essential oil (single or a blend)
2 ml/g vitamin E oil
30 drops plant glycerol of your choice

## Method

Shave the beeswax using a cheese grater until you get three tablespoons of beeswax shavings. Combine beeswax and the

Fat Stage ingredients in a double boiler until all ingredients are melted and the temperature has reached 176°F (80°C).

In your second double boiler, heat the water to the same temperature (176°F / 80°C), gradually adding glycerin and a preservative, if using.

Turn off the heat under both double boilers. Pour the Water Stage ingredients into the melted Wax and Fat Stage ingredients. Pour slowly in a thin stream and continuously whisk the mixture clockwise for five minutes. You can also use a stick blender but please be careful to avoid splattering the boiling hot liquid on yourself.

Allow the mixture to cool naturally without using fans or placing it in a fridge. Stir with a stainless steel spoon or a spatula until the mixture reaches desirable consistency without clumps.

Once the mixture cools to 104°F / 40°C (pleasantly warm to the touch), add all Value Stage ingredients, except essential oils.

When the mixture has cooled to 86°F / 30°C, add essential oils and blend thoroughly.

Pour the mixture into a jar while it's still hot and runny. I find that letting the balm cool down in open jars without their lids closed tightly helps maintain a smooth surface on the cream, which is much more appealing. Closing your lids too quickly may form a vortex (a hole) in the middle of a jar, which doesn't affect the performance of the balm or cream, of course.

If you want to make a balm or an ointment, skip the water or the whole Water Stage completely and simply melt and whisk together the Wax and Oil stages, cool them down to 104°F / 40°C and add all of the Value Stage ingredients.

Stick to the following proportion: one part beeswax to two parts oil. Using less beeswax will produce a highly emollient, thin balm approximately the consistency of Vaseline. Only use a very little beeswax if you plan to make a lip gloss and use a lot more (up to half oil, half beeswax) if you want to make a hair styling wax or a hand balm.

# Common Issues with Natural Moisturizers

Here are some tips that may help you deal with the most common issues that occur when you make your own creams, lotions, and masks. I wish someone had explained these things to me as I was starting my own line of skincare products!

### Did your cream become too runny?

Sometimes this happens if you did not use enough emulsifier. Please make sure to use the recommended amount of emulsifier, and if necessary, refer to the manufacturer's instructions.

### Did your cream come out too thick?

This may have happened because you used too much beeswax or an emulsifier in addition to already solid plant butters. You can add boiling water or cold aloe vera gel to the cream while whisking briskly.

### Did your cream change its color after cooling down?

This sometimes happens if you used hydrosols instead of water. Plant extracts and vitamins, such as beta carotene, may also cause the change in color. There's nothing dangerous about that. Green beauty products can have variations in color due to the unprocessed nature of their ingredients.

### Did your cream grow a yellow or blue crust after a few weeks of use?

This happens due to fungal growth in your product. Bacteria and fungi proliferate in water-based emulsions. Bacteria are invisible, but fungi may appear blue and gray on top of your products. Creams with a higher oil concentration will keep fresh without added preservatives for up to six months, but thin, runny lotions will only keep fresh for a couple of weeks in a refrigerator if you do not wish to use any kind of preservative. Vitamins A, C, E, grapefruit seed extract, and glycerin may help extend the lifespan of your homemade products and add therapeutic value to your moisturizers.

## Does your cream smell unpleasant?

One reason is that some raw ingredients oils have naturally strong scents that may combine to produce an odd aroma. There's nothing wrong with a natural unmasked smell, but if you find it particularly unpleasant, you can try and save the day by adding a few drops of citronella oil into the blend. This oil sometimes helps neutralize offensive odors.

Another reason for an offending smell is that one of your ingredients has gone rancid. In this case you need to discard the whole batch, smell all of your ingredients once again, discard the rancid one, and cook another batch from scratch.

# Crème Galen Cold Cream*

*This cream is made according to the original recipe created by the Roman doctor Aurelius Galenus (AD 129–217). Unlike modern cold creams, Crème Galen is made with beeswax and rose petals for the luxurious scent of fresh roses.*

## Ingredients

5 oz rose water
1 oz unbleached or sun bleached beeswax
6 oz extra virgin olive oil
8 drops rose essential oil
4 drops calendula essential oil
4 drops vitamin E oil
20–30 rose petals (fresh or dried)

## Method

Grate the beeswax. Gently heat the rose water in a glass bowl in a hot water bath. In a separate bowl, combine the beeswax and oil, and then gently heat until liquid. Remove both bowls from the heat and slowly pour the rose water into the oil and wax blend, mixing the cream until it becomes soft and fluffy. You can quickly use a stick blender to achieve even lighter, fluffier consistency. When the mixture cools down, add the essential oils, rose petals, and vitamin E. Stir well. Pour into jars when still liquid.

## Application

Use generously as a cleansing cream or as a face and body moisturizer. Apply with clean fingertips in small upward movements, leave for one minute, and then rinse with tepid water and cotton wool.

## Storage

Store up to nine months in a cold, clean place.

# Oats and Olive Rich Moisturizer

*This cream is good for daily hydration and antioxidant protection for easily irritated, sensitive skin. Oats are soothing and calming, thanks to the high content of anti-inflammatory zinc and magnesium, as well as antioxidant selenium. Olive leaf extract is gaining in popularity as a topical antibacterial agent. Echinacea strengthens the skin's defenses, while calendula soothes and calms.*

## Ingredients

1 oz extra virgin olive oil
2 tablespoons emulsifier (cetyl alcohol)
2 oz aloe vera juice
2 ml/g glycerin
0.5 ml preservative of your choice
25 drops / 1 ml calendula macerated flower oil
20 drops Echinacea extract
1 mg olive leaf extract
2 ml/g vitamin E oil

## Method

Follow the recipe for Basic Natural Moisturizer 1. Add calendula oil, Echinacea, and olive leaf extracts, and vitamin E oil when your blend cools down to 104°F / 40°C. Stir well and transfer to a glass jar.

## Application

Apply twice daily to clean, dry skin, avoiding eye area.

## Storage

Store up to twelve months in a cool, clean place.

# Guardian Angel Protecting Soothing Cream

*This cream works best to provide protection and softening for very dry, tight, fragile skin, possibly after chemical peels or another cosmetic or medical procedure. Castor oil is very emollient and protective; it may help regenerate the skin's surface and help heal any irritations. Olive oil is rich in antioxidant phytochemicals, while cocoa butter helps build a protective layer to shield from the elements. Melissa (lemon balm) is very soothing and cooling.*

## Ingredients

1 teaspoon cocoa butter
1 tablespoon extra virgin olive oil
1 teaspoon castor oil
4g emulsifier
½ cup lemon balm tea
1 tablespoon glycerin
0.5 ml preservative of your choice
25 drops / 1 ml calendula macerated flower oil
2 ml/g vitamin E oil

## Method

Follow the recipe for Basic Natural Moisturizer 1, replacing the boiling water with lemon balm tea. Add oils when your blend cools down to 104°F / 40°C. Stir well and transfer to a glass jar.

## Application

Apply to clean, dry skin, avoiding eye area.

## Storage

Store up to six months in a cool, clean place.

# Eczema Soothing Moisturizer

*This formula offers lightweight hydration for delicate, easily irritated skin with eczema. Evening primrose and rosehip oils are very helpful in preventing and soothing eczema flare-ups, thanks to omega-3 essential fatty acids, especially gamma-linolenic acid. Sunflower oil is very gentle on skin, and the essential oils suggested here help relieve itch and soothe irritation. This recipe deliberately suggests no preservatives, except vitamin E oil and grapefruit seed extract.*

## Ingredients

1 tablespoon sunflower oil
½ teaspoon evening primrose oil
½ teaspoon rosehip oil
4g emulsifier
2 ml/g glycerin
1 cup green tea
10 drops rose essential oil
10 drops lemon verbena essential oil
5 drops peppermint essential oil
20 drops grapefruit seed extract
1 mg olive leaf extract
2 ml/g vitamin E oil

## Method

Follow the recipe for Basic Natural Moisturizer 1, using green tea as a water phase ingredient. Add essential oils, grapefruit and olive leaf extracts, and vitamin E oil when your blend cools down to 104°F / 40°C. Stir well and transfer to a glass jar.

## Application

Apply twice daily to clean, dry skin, avoiding eye area.

## Storage

Store up to nine months in a cool, clean place.

# After Shave Light Moisturizer

*This recipe makes a light moisturizer that is soothing, protecting, and hydrating — great for delicate skin that has been shaved or waxed. Oats are very soothing and calming, thanks to the high content of anti-inflammatory zinc and magnesium, as well as antioxidant selenium. Olive oil is not too greasy, and I use it a lot for my own moisturizers.*

## Ingredients

1 oz extra virgin olive oil
4g emulsifier
2 oz aloe vera juice
2 ml/g glycerin
0.5 ml preservative of your choice
25 drops / 1 ml calendula macerated flower oil
20 drops Echinacea extract
1 mg olive leaf extract
2 ml/g vitamin E oil

## Method

Follow the formula for Basic Natural Moisturizer 1. Add olive calendula oil, Echinacea, olive leaf extract, and vitamin E oil when your blend cools down to 104°F/40°C. Stir well and transfer to a glass jar.

## Application

Apply to clean, dry skin, avoiding eye area.

## Storage

Store up to six months in a cool, clean place.

# Aromatic Balancing Face Lotion

*This lightweight lotion can be used daily under makeup or after shaving thanks to its delicate unisex scent. Calendula strengthens your skin against damaging effects of the sun but does not actually shield from ultraviolet radiation. Sandalwood, tea tree, and cypress essential oils should be used in moderation.*

## Ingredients

½ oz sweet almond oil
3g emulsifier
2 oz orange water
2 ml/g glycerin
0.5 ml preservative of your choice
15 drops / 1 ml tea tree essential oil
5 drops sandalwood essential oil
5 drops cypress essential oil
20 drops calendula tincture or glycerite
2 ml/g vitamin E oil

## Method

Follow the recipe for Basic Natural Moisturizer 1, using orange water as a water stage ingredient. Add more heated orange water if the lotion feels too thick. Add calendula extract and vitamin E oil when your blend cools down to 104°F/40°C. Add essential oils when your blend reaches room temperature. Stir well and transfer to a pump bottle.

## Application

Apply daily to clean, dry skin, avoiding eye area.

## Storage

Store up to nine months in a cool, clean place.

# Green Skin Food

*This recipe makes a cupful of a rich, multipurpose moisturizer without the use of animal ingredients, such as lanolin. Thanks to rosemary essential oil, which also works to rejuvenate and stimulate the skin, this cream will keep fresh for at least three months in a cool, clean place.*

## Ingredients

½ oz extra virgin olive oil
½ oz coconut oil
2 tablespoons jojoba oil
1 oz beeswax
2 oz lavender or rose hydrosol
1 teaspoon glycerin
25 drops / 1 ml calendula macerated flower oil
20 drops rosemary essential oil
10 drops neroli essential oil

## Method

In a double boiler, melt the oils and the beeswax until liquid, stirring constantly. Combine glycerin and hydrosol, heat slightly in a separate pan, then add to the hot oil and wax mixture. Turn off the heat and beat until the mixture cools down. Add essential oils before the cream hardens.

## Application

Apply to clean skin, avoiding eye area, as often as needed.

## Storage

Store up to twelve months in a cool clean place.

# How to Use Facial Oil

Facial oils are more intensive than regular moisturizers. They are best used occasionally, for example, if you have dry skin spells, bouts of acne, sudden onsets of sensitivity, or sunburns. Regular use of facial oils is only recommended if you have dry skin in need of constant added protection. "Dry" oils made with very thin, instantly penetrating oils, such as thistle, hemp, or jojoba, are recommended for daily care for adult oily skin that is prone to acne, yet is sensitive and probably dehydrated due to harsh chemical treatments in the past.

Apply facial oils using gentle outward and upward movements covering your face and neck. If your oil contains not strongly fragrant essential oils, you can try using it around your eyes, but please remove quickly if any irritation occurs. If you use your facial oils in the morning, leave them on for ten to fifteen minutes (or as long as it takes you to eat your breakfast,) tissue off or blot the residue, then apply your regular day cream or sun protection product.

Facial oils are best used overnight. If your facial oil contains any tinted oils or has any orange or yellow color to it, make sure to protect your bed linen with some old towels because stains from essential oils are nearly impossible to remove.

# Sweet Dreams Facial Oil

*This simple recipe was inspired by nineteenth-century beauty guru Harriet Hubbard Ayer. I have added a few other useful essential oils that work really well for dry, lackluster skin at any age.*

## Ingredients

½ oz grape seed oil
25 drops calendula macerated oil
10 drops rose essential oil
10 drops melissa (lemon balm) essential oil
5 drops chamomile essential oil
2 ml vitamin E oil

## Method

Combine all ingredients in a small bottle with a dropper or a pipette application and shake well to mix thoroughly.

## Application

Apply to clean skin, avoiding eye area.

## Storage

Store up to twelve months in a cool, clean place.

# Oily Skin Rescue Serum

*Hemp and thistle oils are perfectly safe for oily skin because they penetrate instantly and do not clog pores. This blend helps rescue oily skin from breakouts, inflammation, and post-acne marks.*

## Ingredients

½ oz hemp or thistle oil
25 drops calendula flower oil (in jojoba base)
10 drops tea tree essential oil
10 drops lemon oil
8 drops thyme essential oil
2 ml/g vitamin E oil

## Ingredients

Combine all ingredients in a small bottle with a dropper or a pipette application and shake well to mix thoroughly.

## Application

Apply to clean skin, avoiding eye area.

## Storage

Store up to twelve months in a cool, clean place.

# Firming Eye Contour Oil

*This formula uses gentle plant oils to help restore and maintain moisture balance around the eyes. Fine non-irritating oils help strengthen sensitive skin and prevent premature aging. Black currant oil can be squeezed from capsules sold as a supplement in many health food stores.*

## Ingredients

2 tablespoons sweet almond oil
2 tablespoons evening primrose oil
1 teaspoon rosehip oil
20 drops black currant oil
1 ml vitamin E

## Method

Combine all ingredients in a small bottle with a dropper or a pipette application and shake well to mix thoroughly.

## Application

Apply to clean skin, avoiding eye area.

## Storage

Store up to twelve months in a cool, clean place.

# Glow Reviving Oil

*This luxurious, fast-penetrating oil is versatile and can be used to nourish your face, hands, and décolleté area.*

## Ingredients

½ cup sweet almond oil
1 drop orange essential oil
1 drop clove essential oil
1 drop jasmine essential oil
½ teaspoon of gold-toned mineral shimmer

## Method

Combine all the oils in a bottle and shake vigorously. Add the mineral glimmer. Shake again to distribute the pigment.

## Application

Shake well before use and apply as often as needed.

## Storage

Store up to twelve months in a cool, clean place.

# Soothing Face Oil

*This antioxidant oil blend comforts irritated, red, or hot skin, especially in winter time or after prolonged sun exposure.*

## Ingredients

    1 tablespoon rosehip oil
    1 tablespoon olive oil
    2 drops calendula essential oil
    1 drop chamomile oil

## Method

Combine all the oils in a bottle and shake vigorously.

## Application

Shake well before use and apply as often as needed.

## Storage

Store up to eighteen months in a cool, clean place.

# Golden Shimmer Lip Balm

*I found that beeswax-based lip balms go stiff and dry on my lips faster than those based on plant waxes. If formulated incorrectly and too little beeswax is melted with too much oil, wax can leave an unpleasant ridge along the lip contour. For this reason I like to experiment with other waxes, like soy and jojoba, which, as an added bonus, make truly vegan lip products.*

## Ingredients

1 tablespoon coconut butter
1 tablespoon soy wax
3 drops vanilla extract
1 drop rose essential oil
1 pinch of shimmery pink mineral blush
1 pinch of pure golden mineral glimmer

## Method

Place the soy wax and coconut butter in a small glass jar, set jar in bottom of a shallow pan; fill the pan with enough water to reach the middle of the glass jar. Heat the pan until the mixture melts. Allow the mixture to cool slightly. Add the rose oil and carefully spoon in the mineral pigments. Add each color one at a time to allow colorful waves of color to form. Blend well with a small spatula and let the balm cool completely before using.

## Application

Apply generously, as often as needed.

## Storage

Store up to twelve months in a cool, clean place.

# Sweet Kisses Lip Scrub

*A lip-smacking, lip smoother made with tasty brown sugar and a heavenly dose of real vanilla! A must-have if you are prone to lip licking in the winter (or kissing on a frosty winter evening). This recipe makes enough product for three months of frequent use, but if you need more of this yummy, scrub, feel free to multiply the recipe.*

## Ingredients

    1 tablespoons fine brown sugar
    1 tablespoon caster sugar
    1 tablespoon jojoba oil
    10 drops vanilla extract
    3 drops peppermint essential oil (optional)

## Method

Combine the ingredients in a small glass jar and give them a really good stir.

## Application

Use as frequently as needed, lightly massage into the lips using circular motions, then rinse off.

## Storage

Store up to six months in a cool, clean place.

# Masks & Scrubs

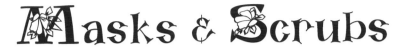

Every now and then, our skin misbehaves—or maybe we misbehave and our skin reacts accordingly? Sometimes we devour too much comfort food loaded with fats and sugars, only to wake up to a nasty breakout (or two). Sometimes our skin faces too much sun, wind, or frosty cold, and a dry, parched complexion is all it has to reward us with. And our skin is especially touchy during that particular period of the month when all we need is lots and lots of chocolate, applied topically as a mask and taken internally as delicious bars and cakes.

Whatever our current skin concern is, masks and scrubs are perhaps the most economical way to deal with a skin disaster. You can prepare a small batch of a mask, store it chilled, and use it daily within a week to see visible results after a short period of time. This can boost your spirit and, in return, boost your skin's glow.

I recommend preparing a large batch of the mask and use it daily to rebalance your skin and bring it back to its usual self. It normally takes a week, but sometimes can take as much as ten days or even two weeks. After finishing the mask, you can return to a normal routine.

The best time to use a mask, of course, is bedtime. This way, you are relaxed and comfortable. The sink and the towel are handy. Ideally, you can try and meditate with your mask on, but you can also read, socialize online, watch TV, or listen to music. Anything goes as long as you don't smile a lot.

Some of the masks are best to use in the morning. If you have a minute or two to spare in the morning, try gently rubbing your face with a scrub. You will be rewarded with a glowing complexion, and makeup will look much prettier. Men can skip the scrub in the morning because they already exfoliate as they shave, but they can use a clay-based mask to soothe and purify the skin.

# How to Make Facial Scrubs

Facial scrubs are made of mildly abrasive particles in a creamy or gel base. They help remove dead skin cells, boost circulation, and stimulate the skin. If you use a scrub regularly every other day for a month, you will notice a much more even, smooth skin texture and much fewer wrinkles and puffy areas. If you combine scrubbing particles with some clay, your preparation will be twice as effective at treating oily problem skin.

Most scrubs can be prepared just from two or three ingredients. Oatmeal, almond meal, fine sugar, fine salt, ground coffee, semolina, and ground rice all make effective and mild exfoliating ingredients. You can combine them with soy or rice milk, plant oils, herbal infusions, green tea, or plain water. Here's a simple procedure to make your supergreen scrubs from scratch:

1. Combine your chosen dry ingredients in a bowl and stir well. You can make this blend (at Petite Marie Organics, we call this an Exfoliating Base) in advance and store in a tightly closed container to use any time you like. I have a few blends that I use frequently. One is a fine sea salt blended with Fuller's Earth clay for my oilier skin days. Another is oatmeal and brown sugar for the body. And yet another one is spirulina, hemp flour, and fine sea salt for my sensitive, dry days, when my skin can use a bit of nourishment combined with a thorough scrubbing action of salt to prevent dry flakes from forming and to help my hydrating facial oils penetrate better.

2. For a single application of your scrub, mix one teaspoon of Exfoliating Base with one tablespoon of liquid base, such as tea, water, juice, or herbal infusion. You can also add a little plant oil to make your scrub more nourishing and suitable for dry skin. Stir well.

3. Apply your homemade scrub in upward, gentle circular movements. Avoid pulling your skin or rubbing for too long

on the same area. Avoid the delicate eye area. If you want to exfoliate your dry, chapped lips using the same scrub, do it using small horizontal or circular movements. Massage your face for two minutes if possible, but not for less than 30 seconds.

4. Rinse your skin and pat face dry; apply a facial toner and a moisturizer of your choice.

# Apple, Lemon and Milk Scrub

*This 2-in-1 mask and scrub delivers a powerful dose of skin-lightening tannins, enzymes, and vitamin C to help achieve an even skin tone.*

## Ingredients

1 apple, peeled and cored
Rind of ½ lemon
2 tablespoons powdered milk or soy milk

## Method

Puree the apple in a food processor, and then add the lemon and the milk. Blend well until smooth.

## Application

Apply all over the face, avoiding eye area. Leave for fifteen minutes, then rinse off.

## Storage

This recipe yields enough product for two applications. If you plan to make more of this mask, please note that it can be stored chilled for no more than one week.

# Olive and Honey Skin Soother

*This mask is excellent to soothe red, inflamed skin suffering from sun burns or chemical exfoliation. It is super-easy to prepare. Do not use if you are allergic to bee pollen.*

## Ingredients

2 tablespoons honey
1 tablespoon extra virgin olive oil
1 teaspoon cornstarch
1 teaspoon dry milk or soy powder (made from whole beans)
¼ cup water or green tea

## Method

Combine all ingredients in a bowl and stir well to achieve a smooth custard-like paste. Add more water or green tea to make the mask thinner.

## Application

Massage the "sauce" into your face and neck. You may cover your face with a warm, moist cotton or cheese cloth mask. Relax for fifteen minutes or longer, then rinse off the mask with warm water.

## Storage

This mask is best used on the day of preparation.

# Lemon Zest, Milk and Almond Polish

*Use this scrub to lighten and brighten a dull, unevenly pigmented complexion. Milk supplies our skin with the skin-firming protein lactose, as well as lightly exfoliating lactic acid. Lemon rind contains antibacterial phytochemicals, as well as circulation-boosting citric acid. Ground almonds mildly exfoliate without damaging your skin. I recommend preparing a batch of this mask and use it daily as a post-vacation treatment course to enjoy a more even-toned complexion by the end of the week. To make this recipe vegan, you can use soy milk for equally great results.*

## Ingredients

½ whole lemon
½ cup whole milk
½ cup ground almonds
3 teaspoons wheat germ oil

## Method

Wash and chop the lemon into cubes. Combine with milk and almonds and make a puree using a blender. Add wheat germ oil and stir more.

## Application

Every morning or evening, apply one tablespoon scrub on your face, neck, and chest and massage well. Let the mask sit on your skin for five minutes before rinsing it off.

## Storage

Store up to one week in a refrigerator.

# Breakfast Yogurt Scrub

*Yeast stimulates the circulation and is rich in vitamin B6, while honey acts as a natural antibacterial agent. You can use any leftover fine cereal for this scrub. Oatmeal, quinoa flakes, and baby rice all work really well to gently exfoliate your skin.*

## Ingredients

2 teaspoons plain yogurt
2 teaspoons fine cereal
½ teaspoon brewer's yeast
1 teaspoon Manuka honey

## Method

Combine all ingredients in a bowl and stir well.

## Application

Apply a thick layer to your face, avoiding the eye area. Leave on for ten to twelve minutes and rinse off.

## Storage

Use the scrub on the day of preparation.

# Sugar Mommy Scrub

*This scrub will leave your skin glowing and well-oiled, not raw and tight. You can use it on your face, hands, and even toes for a pedicure on the run (and on a budget). This recipe yields enough scrub for one generous application to the face, neck, and chest area. To make more scrub, simply multiply the recipe.*

## Ingredients

½ cup fine brown sugar
½ cup olive oil
5 drops rose oil
5 drops vanilla extract

## Method

Combine all the ingredients in a glass bowl or directly in a jar with a tightly fitting lid. Stir well to make sure that the sugar is well saturated with the oil.

## Application

Massage the mixture all over the face and neck for two to three minutes. Rinse with warm water and a washcloth to eliminate the oily residue.

## Storage

Store up to two weeks in a tightly closed container.

# Honey and Blueberries Face Scrub

*Blueberries are packed with antioxidants, as well as vitamin C, while honey is an awesome natural anti-inflammatory, antiseptic substance that works magic on all sorts of blemishes, boils, and zits. Fine sugar exfoliates the dead skin cells even if you apply this scrub as a mask and leave it for a few minutes without rubbing.*

## Ingredients

2 tablespoon honey
⅓ cup fresh or frozen blueberries
1 teaspoon caster sugar
½ teaspoon Matcha (powdered green) tea (optional)

## Method

Wash the blueberries and mash them with a fork. Blend honey, blueberries, green tea, and sugar. Stir well.

## Application

Apply to the skin in a generous layer, covering the neck and décolleté area. Leave to work its green magic for fifteen minutes, and then rinse off with tepid water, using gentle, circular motions.

## Storage

This mask is best used on the day of preparation.

# The Beauty of Facial Masks

Facial masks cleanse, nourish, and stimulate the skin. If daily skincare routine products (cleanser, moisturizer, sun protection) ensure a proper delivery of green goodness to your skin, then masks, scrubs, and facial packs are more of a skin detox that purifies and invigorates the skin, making it more resilient to daily stresses.

Many of the foods found in our kitchens make wonderful ingredients for facial masks and scrubs. They make quick, inexpensive, and most of all perfectly green and sustainable ingredients for spa-quality home beauty treatments.

Here are some of the most common kitchen staples that you can use to make masks and scrubs.

| | |
|---|---|
| Apple | Milk |
| Avocado | Oatmeal |
| Banana | Oils |
| Corn meal | Orange and orange juice |
| Cucumber | Papaya |
| Eggs | Peach |
| Flour | Peas |
| Grape and grape juice | Plum |
| Ground almonds | Potato |
| Ground ginger | Semolina |
| Ground cinnamon | Strawberry |
| Ground rice | Tomato |
| Honey | Vinegar |
| Mango | Yeast |
| Melon | Yogurt |

## Making Natural Face Masks

The process is quite simple: combine all the ingredients in a bowl and stir well to make a smooth, custard-like paste. You can always adjust the thickness of the mask to your liking by adding some water, green tea, rosewater, witch hazel, or any other herbal distillate or herbal tea.

When you have reached the desired thickness, prepare your face. Cleanse your face using a mild natural cleanser and lightly exfoliate with one of the simple peeling creams suggested in this chapter, or you might prepare your skin for a mask using an Exfoliating Cleanser by Petite Marie Organics, which exfoliates using rice grains as you cleanse and remove makeup.

To make the application as mess-free as possible, pat your face dry and pull your hair away using an elastic band or pins. Start applying the mask to your face using tiny scoops and going from the center part (T-zone, or nose, chin, and forehead) towards the cheeks and hair line. This way, if you use the drying clay-based mask, your t-zone will receive the most generous treatment and the mask will remain for longer while more fragile areas will not be dehydrated or over-scrubbed.

With masks, a little goes a long way. As a rule of thumb, one tablespoon of each ingredient (for a simple mask not involving essential oils) is usually enough.

Some masks, especially dry varieties that may be mixed with a liquid medium just before use, can be stored for twelve months. But most often, I recommend using up the mask on the day of preparation. Any mask involving eggs, dairy, fresh fruits, vegetables, or flour cannot be stored for more than 24 hours. Masks containing high concentrations of essential oils, clay, and herbal teas may be chilled and kept for longer.

## How to Apply a Face Mask

1. Tie your hair in a ponytail and pin any loose hair strands so that they do not get messy and oily.

2. Apply the mask onto your cleansed skin, using tapping movements. Do not rub the mask into your skin, even if it is meant to be used as a mask/scrub. Do not drag your skin and keep the mask well away from the eye area.

3. Leave the mask on for the recommended period of time, most often for ten to twenty minutes, depending on the mask. If the recipe calls for it, moisten your face and gently massage the mask in circular movements until it is all creamy again. Rinse off the mask with tepid water, gently pat your face dry, and apply a facial moisturizer or a serum of your choice.

# Honey I Shrunk the Pores Mask

*This recipe delivers a mighty dose of skin toning, astringent, and antibacterial ingredients to help smooth troubled skin and visibly diminish the look of pores. While it's impossible to permanently shrink the pores, regular cleansing with various clays certainly helps to keep them clean and less visible.*

## Ingredients

3 tablespoons kaolin or montmorillonite powder
1 tablespoon natural yogurt
1 egg
1 teaspoon honey
(OPTIONAL)
½ teaspoon gingko biloba tincture
¼ teaspoon evening primrose oil
10 drops rosewood essential oil

## Method

Place the clay into a bowl and carefully add the remaining in-gredients one by one, stirring well to get a smooth paste. Add more water or green tea to make the paste pleasant to apply.

## Application

Apply evenly to clean, dry skin, avoiding eye area. Leave on for ten to fifteen minutes, then rinse off with warm water.

## Ingredients

Store up to three days in a refrigerator.

# Antioxidant Fresh Face Pack

*This rich mask helps protect against premature aging with a power-ful dose of antioxidant phytochemicals that reach your skin directly from the plants in their pure form. Use at least once a week to strengthen your skin against daily environmental aggression. You can use xanthan gum (an all-natural thickener produced by micro-organisms), cellulose gum, or a gelatin-free sauce thickener to prepare a gel base.*

## Ingredients

½ cup water
1 green tea bag
1 ginger tea bag
¼ teaspoon xanthan gum (optionally, cellulose gum)
1 tablespoon wheat grass powder
1 tablespoon spirulina powder
(OPTIONAL)
¼ teaspoon ginseng root powder or ½ teaspoon extract
10 drops ylang ylang essential oil
2 drops rose absolute essential oil

## Method

Boil the water. Place teabags in a cup and cover with a saucer. Leave for five to eight minutes to prepare a strong infusion. Sprinkle the thickener on top and whisk well. Add just enough thickener to make a smooth gel. Add wheat grass and spirulina powders and blend more.

## Application

Apply at least twice a week onto clean, dry skin, avoiding eye area.

## Storage

Keep refrigerated for up to two weeks.

# Tropical Facial Peel

*Enzyme-rich fresh papaya and vitamin C-rich mango are delicious and very beneficial for your skin, as well as your overall health. By adding a dash of lemon juice you leave that nasty blotchiness on your face no chance of survival!*

## Ingredients

½ fresh papaya
½ fresh mango
¼ fresh lemon
1 teaspoon corn starch

## Method

Peel, seed, and cut papaya and mango into chunks. Cut the lemon in chunks, leaving the skin on. Blend all fruit in a food processor until smooth. Add the cornstarch to thicken.

## Application

Apply a thick layer on your face, neck, and chest area. Leave for twelve to fifteen minutes and rinse off. You can use the remaining puree to make a smoothie, but you need to reserve enough fruit before adding the corn starch.

## Storage

Store for no more than one day in a refrigerator (you may wish to make two treatments using this recipe.)

# Banana and Almond Skin Polish

*Bananas are rich in de-puffing potassium and happiness-boosting phytochemicals. Ground almonds gently cleanse and polish off dead skin cells. This mask already smells delicious, but if you add a dash of natural vanilla essence, you'll soothe your nerves in no time.*

## Ingredients

  1 ripe banana
  2 tablespoons almond meal
  5 drops vitamin E (to preserve)
  4-5 drops natural vanilla essence

## Method

Peel the banana and mash it into a puree with a fork. Fold in the almond meal and stir well to dissolve any lumps. Add vitamin E and vanilla essence, stir well.

## Application

Apply a thick layer over your face, avoiding eye area. Leave on for ten to fifteen minutes or until the mixture begins to dry. Using wet fingertips, carefully massage the mask into your skin for one minute, then roll off the remainders and rinse your face well.

## Storage

Store up to three days in a refrigerator.

# Troll Princess Mask

*Spinach is rich in antioxidants and vitamins A, C, E, K, magnesium, copper, zinc, niacin, and omega-3 fatty acids. Banana adds potassium, which helps de-puff the troubled areas. Ginger electrifies the skin cells, and mint helps revive glow and zap any nasty zits that ruin your mood.*

## Ingredients

10–15 fresh spinach leaves or a cube of frozen spinach
5–6 leaves of fresh mint or 1 teaspoon dried mint
½ inch fresh ginger or ½ teaspoon ground ginger
½ ripe banana

## Method

Thaw the spinach if using it frozen. Blend all ingredients using a stick blender.

## Application

Apply to the skin in a generous layer, covering the neck and décolleté area. Leave to work its magic for 20 minutes. Don't forget to take your photo while in this mask! Then rinse off with tepid water using a gentle, circular motions and pat face dry. Now upload the photo on the social network of your choice (optional).

## Storage

Please use on the day of preparation.

# Red Carpet Mask

*Honey is the ultimate skin reviver. Glycerin deeply hydrates by helping the skin retain the moisture. Cucumber helps de-puff the eye and cheek area, while egg whites supply the proteins and tighten the skin as they dry.*

## Ingredients

½ fresh cucumber
2 tablespoons honey
1 egg white
1 teaspoon glycerin
1 tablespoon corn flour or caster sugar

## Method

Peel and chop the cucumber. Combine with remaining ingredients in a food processor and blend until smooth.

## Application

Apply a generous layer to the skin, covering the neck and décolleté area. Leave the mask to work its magic for twenty minutes. Rinse off using gentle circular motions and pat face dry.

## Storage

Please use this mask on the day of preparation.

# Plumpkin Mask

*Pumpkin is rich in zinc, which helps purify an oily, blemished complexion. Pumpkin enzymes also work to gently exfoliate the skin without any abrasive particles.*

## Ingredients

2 tablespoons raw pumpkin
1 teaspoon glycerin
1 teaspoon lemon juice
1 teaspoon tomato juice or ½ teaspoon tomato puree

## Method

Peel and finely grate the pumpkin. Combine all ingredients in a bowl, stir well or blend using a stick blender.

## Application

Apply the mask in a thick layer all over the cleansed face, avoiding the eye area. Leave for ten to fifteen minutes, then rinse off with lukewarm water.

## Storage

This mask should be used on the day of preparation. It cannot be stored.

# Garlic Blemish Paste

*This recipe is inspired by Ayurvedic treatment for skin boils and blemishes. Honey is rich in natural antibiotic agents, while cinnamon increases blood flow to the troubled spot, improves circulation, and provides antibacterial phytochemicals to treat in-flammation in the skin. I have added two other powerful antibacterials that hold the formulation together while making the formulation twice as effective.*

## Ingredients

> 1 teaspoon rice or corn flour
> Juice of 2 garlic cloves
> 1 teaspoon cinnamon
> ½ teaspoon honey

## Method

> Combine ingredients in a small, non-metal bowl and stir really well. You may wish to add more flour if the honey is a bit runny. The paste should be dense and sticky.

## Application

> Apply with a clean spatula to the troubled spot and secure with a piece of gauze and a Band-Aid. Leave overnight.

## Storage

> You can store this mask for up to two weeks in a cold, clean placc.

# Lemon Exfoliating Peel

*Lemon is a gentle skin whitener, brightener, and a great exfoliating agent with antibacterial properties. If your skin can tolerate it, you can use fine sea salt instead of almond meal.*

## Ingredients

> 2 tablespoons honey
> Juice of ¼ lemon
> 1 tablespoon fine sea salt or fine brown sugar

## Method

Combine all ingredients in a non-metal bowl and stir well.

## Application

Apply one teaspoon of the mixture on clean skin and gently massage using circular movements. Leave to penetrate for five minutes, and then rinse off with tepid water. Do not use more than twice a week. This recipe produces enough scrub for two weeks of twice-weekly treatments.

## Storage

You can store this scrub for up to two weeks in a cold, clean place, away from children. Be sure to use a glass container, due to the presence of an acid in the formulation.

# Ayurvedic Turmeric Scrub and Mask

*Women in ancient India used an exfoliating skin cream made with milk, turmeric, flour, and wheat bran. This recipe uses the ancient knowledge enriched with modern vitamins that help brighten your skin. This mask is also useful to help remove signs of premature aging from hands and chest.*

## Ingredients

3 tablespoons wheat, rice, or buckwheat flour
1 teaspoon wheat or almond bran
½ teaspoon turmeric
⅓ cup milk or soy milk

## Method

Combine flour, bran, and turmeric in a bowl, stir well. Carefully add just enough milk to make a smooth paste. Stir well.

## Application

Apply a generous layer on clean, dry skin and leave for fifteen to twenty minutes or until dry. Rinse well with warm water.

## Storage

This mask can be stored for up to one week in a refrigerator.

# Age Spot Treatment

*I prefer to use apple cider vinegar, which not only provides naturally exfoliating alpha-hydroxy acid, namely malic acid, but also a host of trace minerals and vitamins. Onion juice contains a whitening antioxidant called quercetin, which helps even out skin discolorations, spots, and post-acne marks and minor scarring.*

## Ingredients

1 onion
3 tablespoons vinegar
2 teaspoons corn flour
10 drops vitamin E oil

## Method

Peel the onion and either blend it with a stick blender or juice with a juicer. Combine with vinegar in a non-metal bowl. Gradually add corn four until you reach a consistency of a smooth paste. Add vitamin E for nourishment and possibly even quicker face brightening.

## Application

Apply generously over the cleansed face, avoiding eye area. You can also use this mask overnight on troubled spots.

## Storage

Store up to one month in a glass container in a cool, clean place.

# Purifying Aroma Clay*

*Wheat germ powder is a natural antioxidant that truly transforms your complexion, while chamomile and lavender rebalance oil production. Kaolin or montmorillonite (Fuller's Earth) are very beneficial for acne-prone skin.*

## Ingredients

½ cup witch hazel
5 tablespoons kaolin or Fuller's Earth
2 tablespoons wheat germ
15 drops chamomile essential oil
10 drops lavender essential oil
10 drops tea tree essential oil

## Method

Combine all ingredients in a bowl and stir well to make a light, creamy fluid. Transfer the product into a bottle with a pump nozzle.

## Application

Every morning or evening, apply one pump (1 tsp) of the mixture onto your wet face and massage well. Let the cleanser sit on your skin for a minute before rinsing it off.

## Storage

You can store this blend for up to two months in a refrigerator.

# Warm Pumpkin and Honey Mask

*This quick mask feeds your skin with toning, lifting zinc from the pumpkin and soothing, purifying honey.*

## Ingredients

5 tablespoon pumpkin, finely chopped
½ cup water
1 teaspoon honey

## Method

Sautee pumpkin over low heat in water. Stir frequently to make sure that pumpkin doesn't burn. Cook the pumpkin until it is smooth and soft, and then add one teaspoon honey. Stir well. Mash well with a fork and set aside to cool to room temperature.

## Application

Apply to the cleansed face and neck and let set for ten minutes. Rinse with warm water.

## Storage

This mask is best used on the day of preparation.

# Potato and Almond Face Brightening Mask

*Potato is rich in whitening enzymes, as well as vitamin C, which helps lighten complexion. Yogurt contains mildly exfoliating lactic acid. This traditional Eastern European recipe is one of my favorites.*

## Ingredients

> 1 medium raw potato, grated
> 1 tablespoon almond meal
> 1 teaspoon olive oil
> 3 tablespoons yogurt

## Method

Combine all ingredients in a bowl and stir well.

## Application

Apply a generous layer to cleansed skin on your face, neck, chest, and hands. Leave for twenty minutes and rinse off with tepid water.

## Storage

This mask is best used on the day of preparation.

# Nourishing Hand Mask with Honey

*This 2-in-1 scrub and mask deeply nourishes dry, chapped skin on your hands. You can easily make in during a vacation for a quick alternative to a salon manicure. If you don't have fine salt or sugar, fine, clean sand also works marvels as a scrub ingredient.*

## Ingredients

2 teaspoons fine salt, sugar, or sand
1 tablespoon honey
1 raw egg yolk
1 tablespoon full-fat cream

## Method

Combine all ingredients in a bowl and stir well.

## Application

Apply a thick layer to your hands and briskly massage the blend into your fingertips. Put on plastic gloves and relax for ten to fifteen minutes. Remove the gloves and rinse your hands with warm water.

## Storage

This mask cannot be stored. If you replace egg yolk with one tablespoon olive oil, this mask would keep fresh for one week in a refrigerator.

# Whitening Egg and Clay Mask

*This mask helps brighten and lighten the complexion. It is most suitable for oilier skin. Egg white nourishes the skin with proteins, while lemon juice helps brighten the complexion.*

## Ingredients

1 tablespoon Fuller's Earth or kaolin clay
1 egg white
1 tablespoon lemon or lime juice
½ cup green or chamomile tea

## Method

Combine all ingredients except the tea in a bowl and stir well. If the paste is too thick, dilute the mixture with freshly brewed green or chamomile tea.

## Application

Apply a generous layer to clean, dry face. Allow to dry and wash off with tepid water.

## Storage

This mask is best used on the day of preparation.

# Lemon and Yogurt Exfoliating Mask

*This quick mask gently exfoliates without the use of any abrasive particles, so it is good for sensitive skin.*

## Ingredients

1 tablespoon lemon juice
3 teaspoons plain or Greek-style yogurt
1 tablespoon aloe vera juice or honey

## Method

Combine all ingredients in a bowl and whisk until thick and creamy.

## Application

Apply to clean, dry skin, avoiding eye area. Leave on for ten minutes and rinse off with tepid water.

## Storage

This mask is best used on the day of preparation.

# Ozone Aloe Whitening Mask

*When you start using organic fruits and vegetables in your home cosmetics, you will be amazed how rich and vivid the scents are. Experts say that the concentration of antioxidants, vitamins, and minerals is higher in organic veggies, too.*

## Ingredients

½ English cucumber
2 tablespoon aloe vera juice
1 tablespoon honey
1–2 tablespoons cow or soy milk powder

## Method

Peel and chop the cucumber, then puree it with a stick blender. Add aloe vera and honey, and then add just enough dry milk powder to make the mask thicker.

## Application

Apply to clean dry face and leave on for fifteen minutes or until dry. Gently wash off with tepid water.

## Storage

This mask is best used on the day of preparation.

# Cucumber and Egg Mask

*This refreshing mask is recommended for mature skin with large pores. It helps even out skin tone and reduces puffiness.*

## Ingredients

½ large English cucumber
3 tablespoons potato or corn flour
1 egg yolk

## Method

Chop the cucumber and puree it in a food processor. Add the rest of the ingredients and stir well.

## Application

Apply to your face and neck area and leave on for fifteen minutes, and then rinse the mask off with warm water.

## Storage

This mask may be stored in a refrigerator for two days.

# Carrot and Egg Mask

*This is an excellent mask to revive your skin tone and achieve an amazing golden glow without use of a fake tanning product.*

## Ingredients

2 fresh carrots
2 tablespoons potato flour
1 egg yolk

## Method

Peel and shred the carrots, then combine with remaining ingredients and stir well.

## Application

Lie down and apply the mask to the thoroughly cleansed skin, avoiding immediate eye area. Let the mask sit for twenty minutes, and then rinse with warm, then cold water. You can make this mask every day if your skin tolerates it well.

## Storage

This mask is best used on the day of preparation.

# Purifying Mask with Green Peas

*This recipe is nearly two thousand years old. Peas were used for skin care purposes by ancient Romans. Mustard and yogurt add tangy, astringent action.*

## Ingredients

3 tablespoons of fresh green peas
1 tablespoon plain yogurt
½ teaspoon Dijon mustard

## Method

Puree the peas in a food processor, then combine with the remaining ingredients and stir well. If you have oily skin, low-fat yogurt is more suitable.

## Application

Apply a generous layer on clean, dry skin, avoiding eye area. Leave the mask on for ten to fifteen minutes, then rinse off.

## Storage

This mask may be stored in a refrigerator for three days.

# Honey and Turmeric Zit Zapper

*This is a traditional Indian recipe for acne blemishes and other skin discomforts. I recommend using sea salt, which is rich in iodine and anti-inflammatory microelements.*

## Ingredients

1 teaspoon honey
1 tablespoon milk or soy milk
½ teaspoon turmeric
1 teaspoon fine salt
(Optional)
½ teaspoon zinc oxide

## Method

Combine all ingredients in a bowl and stir well.

## Application

Apply with gauze or cotton wool pad to problem areas. Leave on for twenty to twenty-five minutes (or overnight) and rinse off with lukewarm water.

## Storage

You can store this mask for three days in a refrigerator.

# Milk and Yeast Face Lifting Mask

*This is a very simple mask that feeds your skin with antioxidant selenium as well as protein and vitamins, especially the B-complex vitamins. If you are over 30 years old, make this mask twice weekly for two months to see visibly smoother, glowing skin without expensive creams or cosmetic procedures.*

## Ingredients

1 tablespoon dry baker's yeast or ½ oz block of fresh yeast
2 tablespoons of milk

## Method

Combine all ingredients in a bowl and stir well until you achieve a custard-like, smooth cream.

## Application

Apply a thin layer of mask, let it dry, and then apply the second layer, concentrating on the areas that need most firming and lifting (cheeks, chin, and forehead). Leave the mask on for twenty minutes, and then rinse off with warm water.

## Storage

This mask is best used on the day of preparation.

# Cream Cheese Nourishing Mask

*This is a lifesaving mask in winter time. Cottage cheese mildly exfoliates and nourishes the skin with proteins and vitamins.*

## Ingredients

3 tablespoons of full-fat cottage cheese
1 teaspoon avocado oil
1 teaspoon honey
1 teaspoon applesauce

## Method

Combine all ingredients in a bowl and whisk well to achieve a smooth consistency.

## Application

Apply a thick layer on your face and neck. To remove, rinse with warm water. You may follow this mask with a chamomile water or green tea infusion. For best results, apply this mask daily for one week.

## Storage

This mask can be stored in a refrigerator for up to one week.

# Apple, Lemon and Milk Scrub

*This 2-in-1 mask and scrub delivers a powerful dose of skin-lightening tannins, enzymes, and vitamin C to help achieve an even skin tone. This scrub is suitable for all skin types, including very sensitive.*

## Ingredients

1 apple, peeled and cored
Rind of ½ lemon
2 tablespoons powdered milk or soy milk

## Method

Puree the apple in a food processor, and then add the lemon and the milk. Blend well until smooth.

## Application

Apply all over the face, avoiding eye area. Leave on for fifteen minutes, then rinse off.

## Storage

This mask is best used on the day of preparation.

# Rosemary and Honey Skin Soother

*This mask is excellent to soothe red, inflamed skin suffering from sun burns or chemical exfoliation.*

## Ingredients

1 cup green tea
A sprinkle of xanthan gum (less than ½ teaspoon)
2 tablespoons honey
1 tablespoon extra virgin olive oil
3 tablespoons aloe vera gel
20 drops rosemary oil
20 drops vitamin E oil (optional)

## Method

Prepare a cup of green tea. Sprinkle xanthan gum on the tea surface and whisk until a gel forms. Add honey, oil, and aloe vera gel. Continue whisking to avoid clumps forming in the mixture.

## Application

Massage into your face and neck. You may cover your face with a warm, moist cotton towel or cheese cloth mask. Relax for twenty minutes or longer, then rinse off the gel with warm water. You can also leave this gel overnight.

## Storage

Keep this gel chilled for up to one month. If using vitamin E, it can be stored for three months.

# Strawberry and Oatmeal Mask

*Strawberries exfoliate and help lighten the complexion while honey and green tea infuse this mask with powerful antibacterial phyto-chemicals.*

## Ingredients

3 medium-sized strawberries
1 teaspoon honey
1 sachet of green tea

## Method

Mash strawberries. Add the honey and dry green tea from a teabag. Stir well.

## Application

Apply all over your face, avoiding eye area. Leave for fifteen to twenty minutes, then rinse off.

## Storage

This mask can be stored for three days in a refrigerator.

# Warm Orange Veggie Mask

*This warm mask relaxes the facial muscles and promotes blood flow, thus resulting in gorgeously smooth, glowing skin. Sweet potato is rich in puffiness-busting potassium, while carrots supply the skin with youth-preserving beta-carotene.*

## Ingredients

1 medium carrot
1 small sweet potato
1 egg yolk
2 tablespoons of milk

## Method

Steam the vegetables, peel, and mash them. Add milk and egg yolk. Add more milk if needed to achieve a consistency of thick cream.

## Application

Apply the mask while it is still warm. Apply a generous layer to your face and neck (avoiding thyroid area) and cover your face with a towel for optimum results. Leave the mask on for twenty minutes, and then rinse off with warm water.

## Storage

This mask is best used on the day of preparation. It cannot be stored.

# Skin Whitening Mask with Potato

*This is a very simple mask that utilizes the skin-bleaching enzyme catecholase in raw potato. If you suffer from uneven skin pigmentation, apply this mask daily for one month to see great results. This mask must be prepared fresh daily.*

## Ingredients

½ medium raw potato
1 tablespoon milk
1 tablespoon wheat or rice flour

## Method

Finely grate the potato, add milk and flour. Stir well to make a thick paste.

## Application

Apply the mask evenly on your face and leave it for twenty minutes or until the mask dries. Remove carefully with a washcloth and warm water.

## Storage

This mask is best used on the day of preparation. It cannot be stored.

# Sun Care

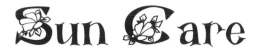

Natural sun protection is my obsession. As someone who faced skin cancer at a very young age, I am extremely careful with my beauty ingredients. I believe in the healing powers of sunshine, I trust my instincts and my common sense, but I know too well that as any powerful medicine, sun can become dangerous when used recklessly and in excess.

Many chemical sunscreen ingredients today are suspected of hormone-mimicking or free-radical damage-boosting qualities. Most chemical sunscreens act by penetrating into the upper skin layers where they transform UV radiation into heat and chemical residue. I surely do not want any of that in my body! I do not want my skin to absorb synthetics, which would run chemical reactions with my body's own ingredients, rendering unknown long-term outcomes. Most sunscreen ingredients have never been tested for long-term safety on humans, and of course not on pregnant women or children. Almost all new chemical sunscreens were introduced five years ago, or even less. Another chemical found in conventional sunscreens, retinyl palmitate, is now considered to be carcinogenic. It may *increase* your risk of skin cancer.

I strongly advocate the use of mineral sun protecting skincare products, also known as sun blocks. These include zinc oxide and titanium dioxide. These white-colored mineral powders work by reflecting sun rays back into the air instead of absorbing them. Basically, sun blocks work as millions of tiny mirrors on your skin, warding off all kinds of dangerous sun radiation.

Titanium dioxide absorbs into the bloodstream and accumulates in bone and soft tissues. Most recently, it was discovered that titanium dioxide nanoparticles induced genotoxicity in vivo (in living tissue), "possibly caused by a secondary genotoxic mechanism associated with inflammation and oxidative stress," scientists in the University of California found (Troullier, Reliene 2009). It seems like titanium dioxide may encourage skin damage and oxidative stress. There is another concern regarding the safety of titanium dioxide. When inhaled, its particles cause cell death in lungs and may contribute to asthma (Hussain, Thomassen et al, 2010). Titanium dioxide has no known benefits to the human body other than cosmetic purposes, and I do not see any reasons to use it in cosmetic preparations, especially if a safer mineral sun blocking component, zinc oxide, is available.

I only use zinc oxide in my sun protection products. Zinc by itself is great for your skin and your overall health. It helps soothe skin inflammation, strengthen your immunity, and may possibly help you deal with such skin issues as eczema and acne. To strengthen skin immunity against free radicals, I always include plant antioxidants, calendula (marigold) extract or oil, coconut oil, and vitamins D and E.

By itself, sunscreen, mineral or chemical, cannot be your sole weapon to prevent skin aging or cancer. Statistics show that countries where people use the most sunscreen also have the highest rates of skin cancer. Sunscreen, mineral or chemical, gives us a false sense of security. We slap it on and bake under midday sun rays until we become crispy brown. But even the most potent sunscreens are rendered useless after a few hours of UV exposure. A great benefit of mineral or natural sun blocks is that they do not absorb sun rays. They simply reflect them back. If you apply them once, they will stay there, rain or shine, or until you rub them off after swimming or exercising. You are covered by an invisible cast of tiny mirrors that reflect sun rays and protect your skin. But you can get sunburns with any sun protection products if you stay under midday sun without any added protection, such as hats, sunglasses, and clothing.

You can layer your mineral sun block to achieve better protection on more exposed areas, such as the nose and shoulders. If you buy an SPF 30 rated mineral sun cream, you can apply it in a thick layer and then reapply in a few minutes to achieve truly remarkable protection. Truth is, whitish residue may be visible, but if your skin is fair, this may even work as a good makeup base or a no-makeup day skin tone evener.

Babies are very sensitive to fragrance, and I suggest avoiding all kinds of scents, natural or synthetic, in all baby care products, including sun products. I know that natural ingredients may not smell as appealing, but I prefer my baby to smell of natural oats rather than artificial roses. Most sun protection products are recommended for use on infants six months upwards. On my little one, I used plain baby lotion mixed with zinc oxide (1 part zinc oxide to 10 parts baby lotion), and she has never had sunburns. Later on, I blended an "adult" version of a simple zinc oxide cream in a pretty bottle for her. This way, she got used to applying a sun cream every day. I have even decorated the bottle with princesses and fairies. Just keep the bottle in the suitcase when you travel, especially if you make more than 100ml of cream at once.

Early childhood sunburns can turn into skin cancer at a very early age. It is *vital* to monitor your baby's moles, freckles, and other skin discolorations. Make it a rule to do a yearly checkup of your baby's and your own skin at a dermatologist.

With physical (mineral) sun blocks, you can get decent protection at SPF 15. This can be achieved by including at least 10 percent zinc oxide in the formulation. After that, many zinc oxide based creams tend to leave a white residue on skin, which turns many people off. To be truly protective, your sun product should bear an index of at least SPF 30. This means that you must add 20 percent or more zinc oxide to your base cream and stir well to avoid lumps.

I believe that your sun block should be appealing and pleasant to use. For most of us, sunscreen application is a chore, and that's why many of us do not care about applying sun protection products liberally and often. I make my own sun protection products packed with antioxidants, so that in summer you would not have to apply an anti-aging product and then top it with a sun protection product and then possibly makeup. Sun protection by itself is an ultimate anti-ager and life-extender, and I make sure mine are packed with everything I want from a good day cream: minerals, vitamins, antioxidants, and probably just a little bit of shimmer! Please note that citrus oils, especially bergamot, are not recommended in sun care products because they may cause photosensitivity.

Here's a tip: always, always wear mineral sunscreen when traveling by air, especially if you sit near the window. You may not get a tan, but your skin is damaged by UV radiation seeping from the windows—and at high altitude you have no ozone layer to protect you.

# Basic Unscented Sun Cream

*This is a really simple, no-frills sun protection cream that should give you SPF 30 or more if you use all the ingredients in the right proportions and stir well to avoid zinc oxide clumps in one place and zero sun protection in another. You must use zinc oxide in concentration of no less than twenty percent to achieve solid mineral sun protection.*

## Ingredients

2 oz Basic Cream 1
1 oz jojoba or sweet almond oil
0.8oz / 24 g zinc oxide
1 oz filtered water
20 drops vitamin E

## Method

Prepare the Basic Cream 1 according to the recipe on page 74. Place zinc oxide into the bowl. Pour the oil on top and stir well to make a uniform mass. Carefully pour Basic Cream 1 on top of zinc oxide and oil blend. Whisk briskly or use a stick blender. Beware of spills, because they can be hard to wipe off.

Add just enough water (but not more than one ounce) to the blend to make a comfortably smooth cream.

## Application

Apply evenly prior to or during sun exposure. Apply the second layer to sensitive areas, such as nose, forehead, and chest.

## Storage

Without added natural preservatives, this blend can be stored for two months.

# After Sun Skin and Hair Repair

*Alexander the Great learned to use the juice of aloe to help heal the wounds in his soldiers during his conquering of Egypt. This cooling, healing gel feels good on your sun-drenched skin, like a glass of water when you are thirsty. Sunflower oil helps prevent skin dehydration, while aloe vera and peppermint cool and soothe.*

## Ingredients

1 cup water
3 tablespoons aloe vera juice
¼ teaspoon xanthan gum
2 tablespoons sunflower oil
15 drops lavender essential oil
10 drops peppermint essential oil

## Method

Combine water and aloe vera juice. Sprinkle xanthan gum over the liquid and stir briskly to prevent lumps from forming. You can also use a stick blender for one to two minutes or until the lumps are gone. Carefully add sunflower oil and blend more. Do not blend for too long, or the gel becomes runny. Add essential oils and stir well.

## Application

Apply generously to the areas of concern. Avoid the eye area.

## Storage

Store up to one month in a refrigerator.

# Sun Saver Antioxidant Serum

*I believe in the health-protecting abilities of the sun, and whenever I tan, I make sure to protect my skin three times: first time, with this antioxidant-rich serum, second time, with a mineral sunscreen, and third time with a potent antioxidant supplement containing lycopene and resveratrol. This serum alone will not protect you from possible premature aging caused by UV radiation, but it will surely strengthen your skin's defenses against free-radical aggression that is thought to be one of the causes of skin cancer. Most of the ingredients in this serum are easily available from health food shops or online.*

## Ingredients

 1 oz grape seed oil
 1 oz linseed (flax seed) oil
 5 drops (3 capsules) beta-carotene
 5 drops pycnogenol (pine bark extract)
 10 drops vitamin E (naturally sourced tocopherol)

## Method

Combine oils in a bottle. If using antioxidants from liquid caps, add them to the mixture. Add the vitamin E oil and shake well to make a uniform blend.

## Application

Apply to clean, dry skin. Follow with a mineral sunscreen in day time.

## Storage

This blend can be stored for up to one year in dark, cool place.

# Organic Body Gloss*

*Whenever my skin feels dull or looks flat and unappealing, I boost its glow with this special oil. If you are generous with mica-based skin glimmer or a shimmer, your legs and arms will glisten with this amazing glossy formula. And if you use organic oils as the base, you will achieve a truly organic body formulation.*

## Ingredients

1 oz olive oil
1 oz castor seed oil
3 tablespoons mica body shimmer (golden is the best)
10 drops vitamin E (naturally sourced tocopherol)
20 drops rose essential oil
5 drops geranium essential oil
5 drops sandalwood essential oil

## Method

Combine the oils in a bottle. Carefully funnel in the mica. If using antioxidants from liquid caps, add them to the mixture. Add the vitamin E and essential oils. Shake well to make a uniform mixture.

## Application

Shake well before use. Apply to clean, dry skin. Tip: if your skin is naturally dark, you may use a deeper shade of mineral powder foundation blended with some pure golden body shimmer to achieve truly natural, luminous results.

## Storage

Store up to one year in a dark, cool place.

# Post-Tanning Scrub for Glowing Skin

*After emerging from the sea, the last thing you think your skin needs is salt. But fine sea salt makes the most amazing skin peeling agent. As you massage this scrub into your skin, salt granules dissolve and become milder, and the risk of over-scrubbing your skin is minimal. Sour cream exfoliates with lactic acid and nourishes with milk proteins and fats. Rose and grapefruit prevent premature aging and smells gorgeous. If you don't have these oils around, feel free to experiment with the ones you've got already, but please keep the concentration to the bare minimum. The following recipe provides enough scrub for a full body application.*

## Ingredients

2 tablespoons fine sea salt
4 tablespoons sour cream
2 drops grapefruit essential oil
4 drops rose macerated oil

## Method

Combine the salt and the sour cream in a shallow bowl. Add the oils and stir well.

## Application

Gently massage the scrub into your skin. Rinse off with tepid water.

## Storage

This scrub must be used immediately before the salt granules have dissolved.

# Sun Protection Beauty Oil

*This beauty oil contains botanicals that help boost the effectiveness of your sunscreen and prevent skin dehydration. Many plants supply our skin with phytochemicals that support our natural sun protection mechanisms. This is the best way to support the skin's own production of melanin. This oil can be used on your face, body, and even hair.*

## Ingredients

½ cup sesame oil
½ cup sunflower oil
1 teaspoon vitamin E
7 drops beta-carotene

## Method

Combine the oils in a glass or plastic bottle and shake well.

## Application

Apply generously and as often as needed.

## Storage

Store up to twelve months in a tightly closed container.

# Skin Protecting After-Sun Mask

*This exfoliating mask helps even out a blotchy complexion resulting from erratic sun behavior. It also helps to lighten your skin if you did not plan to tan. Do not use this mask on sunburned skin or you risk aggravating your skin's condition. I recommend freshly squeezed orange juice to deliver maximum goodness to your skin.*

## Ingredients

    2 teaspoons fine sea salt
    1 tablespoon orange juice
    2 tablespoons aloe vera gel
    1 teaspoon milk
    1 teaspoon rice flour

## Method

Combine orange juice and aloe vera gel with milk. Add salt and rice flour. Stir well.

## Application

Apply using gentle, circular motions. Leave on for two minutes, and then rinse with lukewarm water.

## Storage

You can store this blend for up to two days in a refrigerator.

# 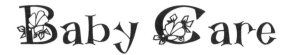Baby Care

Making truly natural baby products was the idea behind Petite Marie Organics beauty line in the first place. Like many new moms, I began shopping for baby essentials the same day as my pregnancy test revealed the crucial second line. I kicked off my stilettos, popped on my ballerina flats, and embarked on a full-time organic shopping spree.

Which led me to a new dilemma (that resulted in Petite Marie line of life) — since most organic baby products are nothing but clever marketing of regular products for sensitive adults, why can't green and savvy moms have the best of baby and mom's skincare in one jar? I applied my homemade stretch mark oil (later evolved into Organic Baby Oil) to my cuticles, face, toes, and, of course, my zeppelin belly. I washed my face and hair with Happy Face cleanser as I was pregnant and I still use it on my petite Marie. When she has a heat rash or skin irritation, I soothe skin with Kiss of Love cream that I have also used on my own face for many years (but then I add a few more real kisses to her area of concern.)

My idea is as follows: parenting is your chance to change your life for the better. This could be the right time to swap your beauty habits for greener ones without spending too much money. Now you can make some essential baby care products for your little one and use them to take care of your skin and hair.

Tip: I prefer to use glass bottles for all baby needs unless I travel and an empty 100ml glass container is not readily available. I know that glass bottles may break when dropped, but this is still a better option than loading the baby product with chemicals leeching from plastic bottles.

As a mom, I can be busy and messy, and still I have managed to break just one bottle in four years of all-glass use in our kitchen and bathroom (and that bottle was dropped by Marie into the toilet — she really needed to make sure it goes BANG!) So don't fret glass bottles, they are much more durable than you think.

# Organic Baby Oil

*Virtually any unscented organic plant oil can be used to moisturize a baby's skin. Avocado, grape seed, and virgin olive oils are among the best. According to scientific studies, babies prefer vanilla to any other scent, so I like to use organic vanilla in all skincare products for children. It is very mild and very rarely causes allergic reaction.*

## Ingredients

½ cup grape seed oil
½ cup olive oil
1 tablespoon wheat germ oil
5 drops vanilla essence or vanilla glycerite

## Method

Combine all ingredients in a bottle and shake well to blend.

## Application

Use this oil generously for baby massage, scalp massage, and, of course, you can use it to moisturize your own skin, mend split hair ends, and groom your cuticles.

## Storage

Store up to twelve months in a cool, clean place.

# Happy Bum Flower Balm

*This is a very emollient yet thin balm that contains no added emul-sifiers, such as beeswax. It glides effortlessly over baby's skin, which is important if you have to deal with rashes and irritations. Eczema sufferers of all ages will love the cooling, lightweight feel of this balm.*

## Ingredients

½ cup shea butter
½ cup coconut oil
12 drops calendula extract
10 drops chamomile extract
1 teaspoon zinc oxide
1 teaspoon vitamin E

## Method

Heat the shea butter and coconut oil in a shallow pan. Do not boil. Remove from heat and stir well; gradually add the rest of the ingredients. Blend until the mixture starts to cool down. Transfer into a glass jar.

## Application

Use as often as necessary.

## Storage

Store up to six months in a tightly closed glass or plastic jar.

# Green Baby Powder

*Sometimes it's unclear whether your baby has diaper rash or a yeast infection. Cornstarch, a popular ingredient in baby powders, can worsen a yeast rash by forming yeast-feeding wet clumps in skin folds. I no longer recommend using kaolin or bentonite in baby products because of their high aluminum content. You can occasionally use these clays for your own masks, but to make baby-friendly skincare products at home, consider using aluminum-free clays. It makes no sense to expose children to neurotoxins at a young age.*

## Ingredients

½ cup baking soda
2 tablespoons montmorillonite clay
1 tablespoon zinc oxide
¼ teaspoon green tea extract (from capsules)
5 drops rose essential oil
5 drops chamomile essential oil
1 sheet of paper

## Method

Combine dry ingredients in a bowl and stir well. Add oils one drop at a time while stirring to make sure that oils disperse completely in the powder. Stir well to avoid any clumps. Make a paper funnel and pour the mixture into a shaker bottle.

## Application

Use as often as necessary.

## Storage

Store up to a year, tightly closed, away from humidity.

# All-Natural Baby Wipes

*Some beauty DIY enthusiasts prefer to make baby wipes from a roll of paper towels, but I found that any old T-shirt cut into squares works much better and is really soft on baby's skin. You can wash and reuse the wipes to be truly green.*

## Ingredients

1 cup purified water
½ cup witch hazel
½ teaspoon calendula extract
2 tablespoons aloe vera juice
5 drops tea tree oil
¼ teaspoon vitamin E oil
20–30 squares of clean cotton fabric

## Method

Blend all the liquid ingredients in a bottle. Shake really well to dissolve vitamin E. Place paper or fabric squares into an air-tight, water-proof container, such as Tupperware. Pour the solution over the pile of fabric squares. Put the lid back on the box and turn it upside down so the solution is absorbed by the fabric and all wipes are properly saturated.

## Application

Use as often as needed.

## Storage

Store up to three months in a container that is tightly closed after each use.

# Skin Clearing Herbal Bath

*This is a traditional European recipe that we used to soothe redness and mild rash in my daughter when she was a newborn. Adults can use this recipe to create a wonderfully soothing and mildly astringent face toner for problem skin.*

## Ingredients

½ cup dried birch leaves
½ cup marigold flowers, fresh or dried
½ cup dried sage leaves
1 pint filtered tap water

## Method

Bring the water to boil, then add the herbs and simmer for ten minutes. Strain into a cup or a larger container.

## Application

Use two cups for one bath and store the rest in the refrigerator.

## Storage

The herbal blend can be stored in a tightly closed container for up to six months. The herbal infusion must be used within two days.

# Soothing Milk Bath

*This blend has been inspired by Burt's Bees Buttermilk Bath Soak, but I did not add any fragrance (who knows what's in it?) and used a few drops of chamomile oil instead. You can use rose oil if you suspect that your little one may be allergic to chamomile (or if this allergy runs in the family). This blend is also suitable for adults with dry, sensitive skin.*

## Ingredients

7 ounces milk or soy milk powder
5 drops chamomile essential oil

## Method

Combine essential oil with powder in a jar and shake well to make sure that the oil completely disappears into the powder.

## Application

To use, dissolve two to three tablespoons in a warm bath. Let your baby relax in the milky water for ten minutes.

# Oatmeal Bath Pouches

*This traditional herbal recipe works to soften your bath water and to soothe and nourish your skin. You can use muslin or pieces of organic cotton for reusable bath pouches. If you are allergic to chamomile, please feel free to skip this ingredient.*

## Ingredients

2 cups traditional oatmeal
2 cups milk powder
½ cup dried lavender flowers
½ cup dried calendula or chamomile flowers
2 drops chamomile essential oil

## Method

Cut small fabric rectangles (the size of this book); fold in half and stitch. Use fabric ribbons to tie the top, which should be the narrow size of the rectangle. Blend all the ingredients thoroughly to make sure that the oil is fully dispersed in the milk and cereal powder. Fill the prepared pouches with the mixture and tie them well with some thread or ribbon.

## Application

To use, immerse one pouch in the bath water and rub it over the baby's skin like a washcloth. You can also use the pouch to scrub your face and body.

## Storage

Store unused pouch in a tightly closed container in a cool, clean place. Keep out of reach of children. Do not reuse pouches.

# 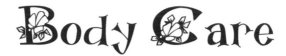 Body Care

The best time to apply body care products is the shower time, morning or evening (or both.) After exfoliating your body with a loofah, a sponge, or a wash cloth, you can either apply a body oil or a body lotion. If your skin needs a bit of revving-up, you can use a generous scoop of a body exfoliating scrub — but make sure to turn the shower off, or your scrub will end up down the drain without having much effect on your skin.

Dairy cream, milk, rose water, and other plant hydrosols make very effective and simple body treatments. You can add a teaspoon of honey or glycerin to make a simple hydrating body mist.

## Healthy Body Skin at Any Age

The skin on our bodies is less prone to aging because it is less exposed to the elements. We usually cover our trunk, neck, arms, and legs with clothes, collars, scarves, and gloves.

A few years ago, when chemical sunscreens were gaining strength and green natural options for sun protection were not easily available, it was common to compare our faces and our bottoms to prove the need to apply a chemical sunscreen every two hours. "Look at your face," salespeople said. It's all wrinkled, parched, and covered with sun spots. And look at the skin on your buttocks, how smooth and taut it is. This is because your bottom isn't exposed to the sun, while your face is.

Now consider this. Our bottom doesn't smile, talk, wear makeup, frown, cry, laugh, eat, and cope with freezing winds and scorching heat. Our bottoms are neatly covered with layers of fabric. The skin on our thighs is naturally four times as thick as the skin on our faces. It does not make any sense to compare faces and thighs when it comes to skin aging. It is the same as to compare cotton socks and leather boots. For unknown reasons, flawed logic of chemical beauty proponents never got questioned.

Just because the skin on our bodies is generally thicker and better protected by our clothes, it doesn't mean we can neglect it and spend all our beauty bucks on our faces and hair. While it's relatively easy to partially reverse the years on your face by using intensive treatments and possible cosmetic enhancing procedures, you cannot do a lot to erase the signs of aging from your neck or your hands.

That's why I suggest applying an anti-aging facial treatment on these fragile areas, starting at the same time when you would start using anti-aging creams or lotions on your face.

Sun spots and wrinkles take years to develop to the point where they become permanent and nearly impossible to remove with natural methods, so it's never too early to spend a minute every day to take care of your neck and hands.

Apply a sun protecting product not just to your face, but to your neck, ears, and hands. Starting at the age 35, I would suggest a weekly anti-aging mask that you would apply to your face, neck, chest area, and hands.

# Creamy Rose Body Mask

*Full-fat cream is especially useful as a body mask when you need to soothe and nourish your skin after sun exposure or when suffering from a sudden bout of itches and rashes.*

## Ingredients

½ cup full fat cream
2 tablespoons rose water
1 teaspoon glycerin
½ teaspoon vitamin E oil

## Method

Combine all ingredients in a bowl and beat well until they form a smooth, creamy paste. Transfer to a jar if desired.

## Application

After a shower, pat your skin dry. Apply with your fingertips in smooth upward strokes over the arms and legs, upwards and outwards over the trunk, and across the shoulders. Apply the second layer over the problem areas. Leave on for ten to twelve minutes, then rinse off.

## Storage

If using vitamin E, store this mask for one week in a refrigerator, otherwise use on the day of preparation.

# Almond and Hemp Body Balm

*Almond and hemp oils are very lightweight and emollient. They are rich in essential fatty acids and skin-nourishing amino acids. Its dark green color and faint nutty smell aren't noticeable when applied to your skin. Warm, deep scents of patchouli and sandalwood complement this balm nicely.*

## Ingredients

5 tablespoons beeswax
1 cup sweet almond oil
½ cup wheat germ oil
½ cup hemp seed oil
10 drops patchouli essential oil
5 drops sandalwood essential oil

## Method

Finely grate the beeswax. Combine with oils in a double-boiler and heat until the wax is thoroughly melted. Stir well. Remove from the heat and continue stirring. When the balm begins to thicken, add the essential oils and transfer to one large glass jar or several smaller jars. Leave the lids open until the balm hardens, or a small vortex may form in the centre of the jar.

## Application

Apply as often as needed to soften and add glow to your skin and hair. You can also use this balm on your toes and cuticles.

## Storage

Store up to twelve months in a dark glass container away from sunlight.

# Sensual Body Lotion

*This fragrant aromatherapeutic body moisturizer is best used in the morning to revive your senses and make your skin glowing and silky smooth.*

## Ingredients

1 cup rose water
½ cup sweet almond oil
½ cup apricot kernel oil
5 tablespoons cetyl alcohol
2 tablespoons sucrose glucoside (optional)
15 drops neroli essential oil
5 drops cinnamon essential oil
5 drops rose absolute (ideally, from Bulgarian rose)
5 drops patchouli essential oil

## Method

Follow the method for Basic Moisturizer 1 as outlined on page 74. Add essential oils when the mixture cools down and feels almost as warm as the human body (becomes pleasantly warm to the touch). Stir well to thoroughly disperse essential oils in the cream. Transfer to a jar or a bottle when the mixture is still warm and can be poured easily.

## Application

Use as often as needed, ideally after showering or exfoliating.

## Storage

Store up to nine months in a closed container away from sources of heat and light.

# Aphrodisiac Massage Oil

*I love massage oils, since they provide the biggest bang for your beauty buck. You can use them to moisturize your skin, to add glow to your hair, to groom your cuticles, and to massage yourself—or a partner, of course! This is a traditional aphrodisiac recipe utilizing ginger, but I have added a fresh modern twist that delights both men and women.*

## Ingredients

3 oz grape seed oil
2 oz sunflower oil
10 drops lemon essential oil
8 drops ginger essential oil
7 drops gardenia essential oil
5 drops jasmine essential oil
5 drops cedar wood essential oil
5 drops patchouli essential oil

## Method

Combine oils in a dark glass bottle and shake well. Leave in a warm, dark place for 24 hours, then shake again. Your blend is ready to use.

## Application

Use as a body moisturizer or for massage.

## Storage

Store up to eighteen months in a dark glass container away from sources of heat and light.

# Warm Vanilla Sugar Body Oil

*This is a perfect blend for winter time, when your skin feels tight and dry because of the lack of sunlight, dry indoors air, and freezing winds outdoors. I suggest using bergamot and other citrus oils in the winter time more freely because they are less likely to cause photosensitivity, unless you tan in a salon, and I hope you do not.*

## Ingredients

½ cup olive oil
½ cup apricot kernel oil
½ cup castor seed oil
1 teaspoon vanilla essence
10 drops mandarin essential oil
8 drops caramel essence
8 drops orange essential oil
7 drops patchouli essential oil
5 drops rose absolute

## Method

Combine oils in a dark glass bottle and shake well. Leave in a warm dark place for 24 hours, and then shake again. Your blend is ready to use.

## Application

Use as a body moisturizer or for massage.

## Storage

Store up to eighteen months in a dark glass container away from sources of heat and light.

# Gentle Body Peeling Treatment

*This recipe suits dry, delicate skin that became flaky and tight after too much sun exposure or winter freeze. You can use this mask on your face, body, and hands, which are often neglected during body care procedures. This treatment helps exfoliate, whiten, and nourish all skin types.*

## Ingredients

4 tablespoons honey
1 lemon
1 teaspoon baking soda
2 tablespoons wheat germ or almond meal

## Method

Warm the honey in a double boiler or bain marie, but make sure not to boil it. Squeeze the juice from the lemon. Remove the honey from the heat and add the lemon juice. Stir carefully. While the mixture is still runny, add baking soda and wheat germ or almond meal. Stir well.

## Application

Apply the warm mixture on the cleansed skin and rub gently. Leave on for ten to twelve minutes if possible. Rinse with luke-warm water and pat your skin dry.

## Storage

Store up to one week in the refrigerator.

# Floral Powder Body Polish

*The traditional simple recipe consisting of sugar and oil is amazingly effective for cuticles, elbows, and knees, but may be a little harsh for delicate skin. You soften the abrasiveness of sugar with ground flower petals and green tea.*

## Ingredients

    1 cup dried rose petals
    3 bags of green tea
    ½ cup fine sugar
    1 cup melissa or lavender water
    ½ cup olive oil
    1 teaspoon sucrose laurate or other cold emulsifier
    10 drops geranium essential oil
    7 drops patchouli essential oil
    5 drops rose macerated oil
    5 drops jasmine essential oil

## Method

Ground rose petals using pestle and mortar. Open green tea packets and empty the contents into a bowl. Combine with rose powder and sugar. Stir well. Add flower distillate, sugar, and cold emulsifier; stir well. Add essential oils and stir more. Transfer to a glass or plastic container.

## Application

Use two to three times a week before or after shower. Apply generously using circular movements, then leave on for fifteen to thirty seconds and rinse off with warm water. Pat skin dry and use your favorite body oil or a lotion. You can make a matching body oil or a lotion using the suggested essential oil.

Make sure you do not exceed the following concentration of essential oils: 15 drops per 3.3 oz/100ml base oil or lotion.

## Storage

This blend can be stored up to three months in a refrigerator or up to two weeks in a dark place in a tightly closed container.

# Tarragon and Verbena Massage Oil for Men

*This blend would make a great gift for any significant man in your life. As with all body oils, this oil has a multitude of uses, from body care to cuticle grooming and, of course, sensual massage. This oil can even be used for shaving, especially if your man has sensitive skin.*

## Ingredients

1 cup jojoba oil
½ cup grape seed oil
1 teaspoon sucrose laurate (if planning to make shaving oil)
10 drops lemon essential oil
8 drops verbena essential oil
8 drops vetiver essential oil (optional)
7 drops cedar wood essential oil
6 drops lavender essential oil
5 drops bergamot essential oil
2–3 stems fresh tarragon

## Method

Rinse tarragon and dry carefully with a towel. Carefully insert it into a clean, dark glass bottle. Add all remaining ingredients and shake gently. Place in a warm, dark place for 24 hours to infuse. Your oil is ready for use or giving away as a gift.

## Application

Use generously to take care of skin, hair, and nails.

## Storage

Store up to twelve months away from heat and sunlight.

# Lemon and Vinegar Foot Soak

*Lemon by itself is extremely effective in getting rid of skin discolorations, flaking, rough areas, and unpleasant smells. By adding apple cider vinegar and skin-softening salt, we prepare a great bath that would make a pedicure a snap.*

## Ingredients

A small basin (approximately 10 cups) moderately hot water
1 cup apple cider vinegar
½ cup sea or table salt
2 lemons

## Method

Pour the water into a bowl. Add vinegar and the salt. Stir well. Squeeze the juice from lemons into the bowl. Add the lemon zest to the water.

## Application

Place your feet into the water and relax for ten to fifteen minutes. When the water cools down, take your feet out, pat them dry, and continue with exfoliation and cuticle treatments.

## Storage

Cannot be stored, must be used on the day of preparation.

# Lemon and Fennel Skin-Firming Gel

*Sweet fennel and juniper are said to encourage toxin elimination and improve circulation in the skin. This helps to smooth the skin surface and eliminate unsightly bumps often associated with cellulite. With daily use, the skin begins to look taut and firm.*

## Ingredients

3 oz water
½ teaspoon xanthan gum
20 drops lemon oil
10 drops sweet fennel essential oil
8 drops juniper essential oil

## Method

Pour the water in a bowl. Measure xanthan gum and sprinkle the powder over the water, whisking briskly. You can use a stick blender if the mixture gets lumpy. Do not blend more than necessary or you will introduce too much air into the gel. Add essential oils and stir well.

## Application

Apply to the problem areas after shower.

## Storage

Store up to three months in a cool, clean place.

# Coffee Cellulite Mask

*Coffee is a strong diuretic, and its topical application helps flush the retained water in the skin, which is often the cause for bumpy, uneven skin texture. Ground coffee makes an excellent exfoliating scrub. You can utilize used coffee grounds for this application.*

## Ingredients

1 cup water
5–6 tablespoons ground coffee
1 teabag of green tea
10 drops grapefruit essential oil
8 drops juniper essential oil
Elastic bandage or plastic film

## Method

Pour the water in a bowl. Add the coffee and the contents of the teabag. Stir well. Add the essential oils and stir more.

## Application

Apply to the problem areas and cover with an elastic bandage or plastic film. Leave on for 15 minutes, and then rinse off.

## Storage

This mask must be used on the day of preparation.

# Honey and Sesame Cuticle Restoring Balm

*This pleasant-smelling balm is great not just for cuticles, but also for lips and other dry, chapped, or coarse skin areas. You can also pack it into small tins or plastic jars and give away as gifts.*

## Ingredients

5 tablespoons grated beeswax
5 tablespoons sesame oil
1 tablespoon honey
1 teaspoon vanilla essence
¼ teaspoon vitamin E oil

## Method

Melt the beeswax and oil in double boiler. Add honey and carefully stir until dissolved. Add vanilla essence and stir more. Pour into containers when the mixture is still hot.

## Application

Rub well into cuticles to soften them and prevent cracking. You can also use this balm on your lips and other dry skin areas.

## Storage

Store up to twelve months.

# Green Eau De Toilette

*To flex your perfumer's muscle, start with one or two essential oils and add more as you gain experience. Don't forget to carefully record the amount of each essential oil you used, so that you can recreate or refine the formula. It's best to use good-quality vodka that will be devoid of any scent.*

*Please make sure you have reached the legal drinking age for your country before you purchase ingredients for this recipe.*

## Ingredients

1 oz vodka
2 tablespoons distilled water
10–15 drops of essential oils of your choice

## Method

Combine vodka and essential oils in the container. Shake well and leave to synergize for two days. Slowly add the distilled water, shaking well. Let the mix sit and synergize for two days or more, if you want a more potent mix.

## Application

Apply as often as needed. Avoid spraying around the eye area or on freshly shaven skin; avoid mucous membranes. Do not take internally.

## Storage

Store up to twelve months in a tightly closed container.

# Carmelite Water (Eau De Carmes)

*This cologne was originally made by Carmelite nuns in France for use as a medicine. The original recipe includes over a dozen herbs and the preparation no doubt involved singing Gregorian chants. Here's a simplified version of this legendary cologne. You may substitute lemon balm leaves with 5 drops citronella oil, but the fragrance will lack the spicy, green scent of dried plants.*

## Ingredients

3 cups vodka
1 cup distilled water
1 cup dried lemon balm leaves
½ cup fresh lemon zest
1 cup dried angelica leaves
1 tablespoon coriander seeds, lightly crushed
1 nutmeg, grated
2 teaspoons cloves
3 cinnamon sticks, crushed

## Method

Place all the spices and herbs in a glass jar, and then pour in the vodka. Close the lid and shake vigorously. Leave in a warm place away from direct sunlight for up to ten days, shaking at least once a day. Strain through muslin cloth, then siphon through a coffee filter into a dark glass bottle with a spray topper. Dilute to the strength you want by adding filtered or distilled water.

## Application

Apply as often as needed, avoiding eye area and mucous membranes.

## Storage

Store up to twelve months.

# Aphrodisiac Solid Perfume

*In ancient times, perfumes were mostly plant-based. Some of the most popular ingredients in ancient Rome were cinnamon, myrrh, jasmine, quince, laurel, jasmine, and rose, which were soaked in oil and gently heated. Remember not to exceed the recommended amounts of essential oils, or you risk irritating your skin.*

## Ingredients

4 tablespoons beeswax
4 tablespoons jojoba oil
2 drops jasmine essential oil
2 drops ylang ylang essential oil
2 drops vanilla extract
1 drop sandalwood essential oil
1 drop rose essential oil

## Method

Gently heat the beeswax and oil in a small saucepan until the wax is melted. Remove from the heat and stir in the essential oils. Pour the mix in a clean lip balm container, a vintage silver pillbox, or any other pretty container with a tightly fitting lid. Let the mixture cool before applying it to your skin.

## Application

Soften balm with fingertips and apply to pulse points.

## Storage

You can store this product for up to nine months in a closed container. Replace the lid promptly after each use to prevent essential oils from evaporating.

# Green Spice Deodorant

*This is a unisex fresh herbal scent that works to neutralize your body odors, rather than masking them or blocking your perspiration completely.*

## Ingredients

1 cup grain alcohol
1 cup witch hazel
10 drops tea tree essential oil
10 drops citronella essential oil
5 drops juniper essential oil
5 drops lemon essential oil
(OPTIONAL)
5 drops liquid emulsifier, such as sucrose laurate

## Method

Combine all the ingredients in a sterilized pump-lid bottle, shake well, and leave in a warm place for one day. Shake well before each use. If you use an emulsifier, the liquid may appear milky. This is perfectly normal.

## Application

Apply as often as needed.

## Storage

Store up to twelve months in an airtight container.

# Natural Clay Deodorant

*This deodorant acts as a very mild antiperspirant by absorbing sweat and trapping it in the clay's porous particles. Make sure you use aluminum-free clay, such as montmorillonite (Fuller's Earth).*

## Ingredients

3.3 fl oz witch hazel
2 tablespoons baking soda
1 tablespoon montmorillonite clay
10 drops citronella essential oil
10 drops tea tree essential oil
10 drops sage essential oil
5 drops lemon essential oil

## Method

Pour witch hazel into a spray bottle; funnel in the baking soda and the clay. Shake well. Add the essential oils if using.

## Application

Shake well before use. Spray generously under arms.

## Storage

Store up to nine months in an airtight container.

# Refreshing Herbal Body Spray

*This recipe is inspired by a natural deodorant line by Weleda. However, I found that none of the scents I have tested work truly effectively for more than two hours on a moderately hot summer day. This recipe combines some of the most effective odor neutralizers that you can blend together in a few minutes and for much smaller cost than most deodorants in a health food store. This recipe yields enough product to take you through two to three months of daily use. A hint: use this spray to disinfect your hands and surfaces.*

## Ingredients

1 cup witch hazel
1 cup grain alcohol (such as vodka)
20 drops tea tree essential oil
20 drops eucalyptus essential oil
10 drops lemongrass essential oil
10 drops benzoin essential oil

## Method

Combine all ingredients in a spray bottle and shake well. Leave to infuse in a warm dark place for 24 hours, shaking the bottle occasionally. The oils may pool near the top; this does not affect the performance of the product. Regular shaking may help disperse the oils. If this bothers you, consider adding a few drops of a natural emulsifier, such as sucrose laurate or glycerin.

## Application

Spray generously to combat odors. Avoid spraying on freshly shaven skin.

## Storage

Store up to two years in an airtight container with a spray nozzle.

# Herbal Insect Repellant Spray

*I found that this super-easy bug spray works non-stop for three to four hours without the need to reapply, and you can spray it on clothes, bedding, curtains, and patio furniture. The essential oil blend can be mixed with a little carrier oil and added to aroma lamps. You can also pour into a handy rollerball container to carry around.*

## Ingredients

3–5 fresh or dried bay leaves
5–6 clove pods
2 cups canola or soy bean oil
15 drops rosemary essential oil
10 drops lavender essential oil
10 drops thyme essential oil
8 drops sage essential oil
8 drops geranium essential oil
7 drops peppermint essential oil
10 drops carnation essential oil (optional)

## Method

Place bay leaves and clove pods in a spray bottle. Pour the base oil on top and then carefully add essential oils. Carefully shake. You can use the blend immediately, but it's best to leave it to infuse for 24 hours.

## Application

Apply evenly on desired surfaces, avoiding eye area. Massage well into the skin. To use in an aroma lamp, combine the essential oil blend with three tablespoons of oil.

## Storage

Store up to eighteen months in an airtight container with a spray nozzle.

# Soda and Myrrh Mouthwash

*In ancient times, soda bicarbonate mixed with myrrh essence was used to cleanse the teeth and keep the gums healthy. Twigs and leaves were used instead of toothbrushes. To prepare more of this mouthwash, feel free to multiply the recipe.*

## Ingredients

2 cups water
2 peppermint teabags
1 cup witch hazel
1 tablespoon baking soda (sodium bicarbonate)
1 teaspoon glycerin
10 drops myrrh essential oil

## Method

Boil the water. Place teabags into a beaker glass and pour the water on top. Let the tea infuse for five to six minutes, then remove the teabags and discard them. Combine with the remaining ingredients and stir well. Transfer to a container.

## Application

Shake well before use. Every morning and evening, rinse your mouth with ¼ cup of the mouthwash.

## Storage

This blend can be stored for up to six months in a closed container. Please replace the lid promptly after each use.

# Hair Care

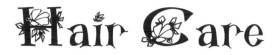

Our hair is an amazing organ with amazing reproductive capabilities. Even when plucked completely, the hair follicle will grow out again. It is a common belief that the strength, quantity, and color of our hair greatly depend on heredity. Still, we are able to influence these matters with proper hair care and supplementation. Premature grayness of hair may be delayed with regular supplementation of B group vitamins. Dandruff and dry scalp can be prevented and cured with essential fatty acid and silica supplementation. Hair growth can be restored with biotin and silica.

Gentle cleansing is the most important step to a healthy crown of hair at any age. However, on our quest to green beauty we are reluctant to replace conventional shampoos with green ones. And often for good reason, because most so called "organic" brands unfortunately load their products with sulfate detergents, synthetic preservatives, and artificial fragrances. Here are the top ingredients to avoid in "greenwashed" hair care products:

- Sodium/Ammonium Lauryl/Laureth Sulfate

- Diethanolamine/Triethanolamine (cocamide DEA is often used in greenwashed products)

- Diazolidinyl Urea/Umidiazolidinyl Urea

- Mineral Oil

- Propylene Glycol/Polyethylene Glycol (PGs and PEGs)

- Phenoxyethanol

- PVP/VA Copolymer (often found in hair styling products)

- Steralkonium Chloride (often used in hair conditioners)

- Parabens (often listed as Germaben and Germall)

To make informed choices, you must be willing to read ingredients labels. Refuse to settle for greenwashed offerings because they undermine the trust in organics and aren't better for the environment than conventional cosmetics.

If you want a truly natural green product, you will be surprised that it is often easier to make one yourself than to scour health food stores and online vendors. This chapter includes easy-to-make shampoos, conditioners, hair treatments, and rinses that are very budget- and environment-friendly.

# Egg and Lemon Shampoo

*This recipe has been adapted from a simple shampoo recipe at CreativeHomemaking.com. I found the original version to be suitable for very dry, fragile hair, due to its very high oil content. I recommend using only egg yolks for hair care, because egg whites take ages to remove from hair. My version suits most hair types, and you can adapt it to your needs by varying the amount of Castile soap in the formulation.*

## Ingredients

1 egg yolk
½ oz olive oil
½ oz Castile soap
1 tablespoon lemon juice
½ teaspoon apple cider vinegar

## Method

Stir egg yolk with olive oil. Carefully combine with the rest of the ingredients in a tall beaker glass. Stir slowly yet thoroughly.

## Application

Wet your hair and use the mixture as regular shampoo. Massage your hair well and leave on for 30 seconds or more before rinsing off with lukewarm water.

## Storage

You can store this shampoo for up to one week.

# Orange Hair Glosser

*Glycerin forms a fine layer on the hair, sealing the cuticle and attracting moisture from outside. This quick and easy toner helps add light moisture to dry, frizzy locks and scalp.*

## Ingredients

1 oz orange water
2 teaspoons glycerin

## Method

Combine both ingredients together and shake well. Transfer to a spray bottle.

## Application

To use, apply daily on towel-dried hair and style as usual. Apply as often as needed.

## Storage

Store up to three months.

# Bugs Away Purifying Hair Spray

*This handy hair mist can be packed in cute colored plastic spray bottles and applied fearlessly any time your little one's hair is in trouble, since this formula contains absolutely no toxic chemicals.*

## Ingredients

  1 cup juniper berry hydrosol / very strong black tea
  2 tablespoons glycerin
  ½ teaspoon cold emulsifier, such as sucrose laurate
  30 drops tea tree essential oil
  20 drops eucalyptus essential oil
  15 drops cloves essential oil
  8 drops peppermint essential oil

## Method

Combine all ingredients in a spray bottle and shake well.

## Application

Shampoo the hair and comb it well. Shake the bottle. Divide the hair in sections and mist the roots generously with the mist. Leave on for two to three minutes, and then comb the hair well with a special nit comb. This mist can also be used to prevent bug infestation after shampooing but before drying the hair.

## Storage

Store up to twelve months in an airtight container with a spray nozzle.

# Dry Scalp Treatment Mask

*This rich, emollient mask helps soothe irritated dry scalp and pre-vent or treat itchy, flaky scalp. Castor oil is believed to promote hair growth.*

## Ingredients

1egg yolk
1 tablespoon castor oil

## Method

Beat both ingredients together until smooth.

## Application

Apply to clean, towel-dried hair. Massage gently into the scalp and leave on for ten to fifteen minutes. Rinse off with warm water.

## Storage

This mask is best used on the day of preparation. It cannot be stored.

# Carrot Top Red Hair Color Reviver

*Carrots are high in vitamin A in its natural form, beta-carotene. This pro-vitamin is naturally red in color and is highly pigmented. Honey provides your hair with strengthening enzymes and minerals, while cranberry acts as a natural penetration enhancer, thanks to the high content of fruit acids. This mask works well for naturally red or auburn hair.*

## Ingredients

2–5 large carrots, depending on the length of your hair (2 for short, 3 for shoulder-length hair, and 5 or more for long hair)
½ cup cranberries, fresh or frozen
1 tablespoon honey

## Method

Wash, scrub, chop, and steam the carrots. Mash with a fork or a stick blender. Add cranberries and mash more. Add the honey and stir well.

## Application

Shampoo your hair and squeeze out the excess liquid. Apply the mask generously over your hair, covering well from roots to ends. Cover your hair with a shower cap and wrap your head with a towel. Relax for ten to fifteen minutes, then rinse off the mask to reveal a glistening crown of hair! Style as usual.

## Storage

This mask must be used on the day of preparation.

# Apple Hair Shine Restoring Mask

*To revive dry, dull hair, all you need is one big apple. This mask also solves dry scalp problems, such as itchiness and flakes. You can also use two or three medium sized apples, depending on your hair length. Choose only fresh apples without any dents or flaws.*

## Ingredients

1–2 large or 3–4 medium apples
2 tablespoons apple cider vinegar
1 teaspoon lemon juice
1 tablespoon corn flour

## Method

Peel, core, and grate the apples. Combine the pulp with the remaining ingredients and stir well.

## Application

Spread the mixture over dry unwashed hair and leave on for twenty to thirty minutes. You can cover your hair with a shower cap or PVC-free food film and then wrap it with a towel. Rinse the mask off with tepid water and follow with a mild shampoo, if desired.

## Storage

This mask cannot be stored and must be used on the day of preparation.

# Avocado and Cucumber Soothing Scalp Treatment

*This hair treatment is a great help if you have a dry, itchy scalp. Cucumber soothes and moisturizes while feeding your hair shafts with strengthening silica.*

## Ingredients

½ large cucumber
1 avocado
1 tablespoon honey
¼ cup water

## Method

Chop the cucumber with its skin on. Peel the avocado. Puree the cucumber and the avocado in a food processor. Otherwise, grate the cucumber and mash the avocado with a fork. Add the honey and dilute with water to make a paste.

## Application

After shampooing and towel-drying your hair, apply the puree all over your head and massage gently into the scalp. Cover your head with a shower cap and wrap it in a towel. Leave on for fifteen minutes and rinse off.

## Storage

Store up to three days in a refrigerator. You can extend the shelf life of this treatment up to one month by adding 1% vitamin C powder (not suitable for sensitive scalps) or vitamin E oil (good for all hair conditions, including very dry and sensitive hair.)

# Banana Cookie Anti-Dandruff Scalp Treatment

*Bananas feed the hair and scalp with vitamin C, potassium, and vitamin B6, while oats are highly absorbing and calming. In fact, colloidal oatmeal is clinically proven to soothe dry, itching scalp. Nutmeg is naturally antiseptic and helps relieve itchiness.*

## Ingredients

½ cup finely ground oatmeal
1 cup water
1–2 very ripe bananas
½ teaspoon ground nutmeg

## Method

Finely grind oats in a coffee grinder or blender. Boil the water and pour over the oats. Let it stand for half an hour. Meanwhile, peel and mash bananas with a fork. Combine the puree with oatmeal and stir well. Add more warm water if needed. Add the nutmeg and stir more.

## Application

Shampoo your hair and squeeze the excess liquid. Apply the mask generously over your hair, massaging it deeply into the roots. Cover your hair with a shower cap and wrap your head with a towel. Relax for fifteen to twenty minutes, then rinse off the mask.

## Storage

This mask must be used on the day of preparation.

# Herbal Hair Strengthening Rinse

*This hair conditioning rinse is suitable for all hair types. It leaves hair glossy and bouncy while diminishing itchiness, scalp dryness, and preventing dandruff. Regular use may help promote hair growth. All ingredients can be purchased in health food stores or online at reputable herbalists.*

## Ingredients

2 tablespoons dried chamomile flowers / 3 chamomile tea bags
2 tablespoons dried peppermint leaves / 4 peppermint tea bags
3 tablespoons dried nettle or 4 nettle tea bags
3 tablespoons dried burdock root
3 tablespoons dried birch leaves

## Method

Place all herbs into a thermal flask and carefully fill it with boiling water. Close the lid and leave the herbs to infuse for two to three hours. Strain the liquid into a glass or plastic container.

## Application

Shampoo your hair as usual and squeeze out excess water. Make sure that your herbal infusion is mildly warm before application. Carefully pour one cup of the herbal rinse on your hair, massaging it well to evenly distribute all over the scalp and to enhance its penetration. Do not rinse. Towel-dry your hair again and style as usual.

## Storage

Can be stored in a closed container for up to one year.

# Coconut Hair Glossy Crème

*This cream imparts a healthy glow to dull, frizzy hair with brittle ends. It can also be used to deeply moisturize the scalp and skin. It is most suitable for dry, chemically treated, or coarse hair.*

## Ingredients

½ ounce cetyl glucoside (check other emulsifiers)
3 oz coconut oil
1 oz olive oil
1 oz  sweet almond oil
1 oz geranium distillate or plain water

## Method

Combine cetyl glucoside with the oils. Heat mixture gently until it is transparent and the emulsifier has dissolved completely. In a separate bowl, heat the distillate (or water) until almost boiling. Carefully add water to the oils and emulsifier mixture and whisk briskly until soft and completely smooth. Transfer to the container of your choice when the mixture is still warm.

## Application

When using as a split end conditioner, massage into hair ends after shampooing and then style as usual. When using as a treatment for frizzy hair, apply to your palms, rub them gently together, and then distribute the gloss along the hair; style as usual. When using to add gloss and definition, apply to dry hair sparingly with your fingertips.

## Storage

Store up to twelve months in a dark glass or plastic container.

# Nutritious Argan Hair Gloss

*Argan oil is perhaps the most promising newcomer in natural hair care. It is lightweight, does not make hair limp or heavy, and imbues an amazing glow and shine even to the most coarse, frizzy hair. While argan oil is still not easy to come by, several reputable suppliers of good-quality natural ingredients offer this amazing oil in small quantities — just enough for your personal use. If you have trouble locating argan oil, which can be used neat or fragranced with a few drops of lavender or geranium oil, the following blend comes pretty close.*

## Ingredients

½ cup jojoba oil
2 tablespoons evening primrose oil
1 teaspoon thistle/sunflower oil
10 drops lavender essential oil (optional)
5 drops geranium essential oil (optional)
5 drops may chang essential oil (optional)

## Method

Combine all ingredients in a spray bottle and shake well.

## Application

Apply a few pumps directly onto the hair or spray onto palms and rub them to warm up the oils. Apply to the areas of frizziness, comb well, and style as usual. Also useful as an occasional hair treatment after sun exposure or swimming in a pool.

## Storage

Store up to twelve months in a plastic or glass container.

# Tea and Jasmine Solid Shampoo

*This all-natural, sulfate-free shampoo is inspired by LUSH solid shampoos, which are very handy if you travel a lot but unfortunately contain just too many chemicals. Original LUSH shampoo tins are made of aluminum, which can leach into the product, but any plastic soap box would work just fine. You can use a special soap mould or you can try a silicone cookie mould. If you plan to give away this solid shampoo as a gift, you can decorate it with some mineral glitter. To make more shampoo, simply multiply the recipe.*

## Ingredients

3 oz melt-and-pour olive or goat milk soap base
2 tablespoons glycerin
1 tablespoon olive, jojoba, or sunflower oil
1 teaspoon fine sea salt
1 teaspoon matcha green tea powder
10 drops jasmine essential oil
5 drops rose absolute or 10 drops rose macerated oil
5 drops tea tree oil

## Method

Melt the soap base according to the instructions. Stir well to avoid lumps. Add glycerin, oil, and sea salt. Stir well. When the soap cools down to lukewarm temperature, add green tea powder and essential oils. Transfer to a soap or a cookie mould. Let cool and remove.

## Application

Rub the solid shampoo into the wet hair and massage well, then rinse. This shampoo is rich and nourishing, so you may not need a conditioner afterwards.

## Storage

Store up to twelve months in a closed container. Please keep the shampoo dry. After use, remove excess water from the jar; leave it open to let the shampoo dry naturally before closing the jar, or you risk ending up with a jar full of soap mush.

# Aromatherapeutic Dry Shampoo

*Dry shampoos work by absorbing excess oils from the scalp and hair roots, making hair less flat and creating more volume and bounce. Most dry shampoos on the market use talc and artificial fragrances. This natural version is based on a time-tested recipe and smells equally appealing to men and women.*

## Ingredients

> 3 tablespoons kaolin (white clay)
> 3 tablespoons corn starch
> 2 tablespoons potato or gram flour
> ½ teaspoon ginger powder
> ¼ teaspoon ground sage

## Method

Combine all ingredients in a bowl and stir to distribute spices well. Transfer into a sifter jar.

## Application

Divide your hair and sprinkle onto the scalp and into the hair roots. Brush your hair thoroughly, and then blow your hair with a hairdryer on cool setting to remove the powder.

## Storage

Store up to one year in a closed container.

# Rose and Mayonnaise Warm Hair Pack

*Mayonnaise by itself is a gorgeous hair conditioner. It has eggs and cream to nourish and moisturize, vinegar to get rid of skin flakiness, and olive oil to revive glow and nourish the hair shaft. Rose transforms this humble product into a luxurious mask, and clay helps absorb excess oiliness.*

## Ingredients

½ cup mayonnaise
10 drops rose macerated oil
2 tablespoons white clay

## Method

Warm up the mayonnaise in a shallow bowl placed in a larger bowl with boiling water. Carefully add the oil and the clay. Stir well.

## Application

Apply generously onto the hair and lightly massage. Cover the head with a shower cap and wrap it in the towel. Leave the mask on for 30 minutes, then rinse off and either shampoo or style your hair as usual.

## Storage

This mask can be stored for up to two weeks in a refrigerator.

# Apple and Sea Salt Scalp Purifying Mask

*Apples are mildly astringent and exfoliating, which helps clarify the scalp and get rid of flaky, dry skin. With regular use, you may relieve itchiness and prevent dandruff. An apple a day keeps dandruff away!*

## Ingredients

1 cup applesauce
2 tablespoons dry milk
1 teaspoon fine sea salt
10 drops tea tree essential oil (optional)

## Method

Combine all ingredients in a shallow bowl and stir well.

## Application

Apply to dry hair before shampooing. Massage the mask well into the scalp and leave on for ten to fifteen minutes. Rinse off and follow with a mild shampoo as usual.

## Storage

This mask must be used on the day of preparation.

# After Sun Hair Restoring Treatment

*This lightweight hair oil is a wonderful styling aid, as well as an emergency treatment should you have overdone it with sun, salt, and wind. Please note that citrus oils should not be used on your skin prior to sun exposure, however, they smell wonderful and work hard to restore your hair to its silky perfection.*

## Ingredients

½ cup jojoba oil
½ cup sunflower oil
10 drops orange oil
5 drops mandarin oil
5 drops neroli essential oil

## Method

Combine all ingredients in a spray bottle and shake well. Leave for one day in a dark place for oils to infuse.

## Application

Spray liberally on your hair after sun exposure. Do not rinse. Style as usual. Can also be used to mend split ends.

## Storage

Store up to eighteen months in a closed container.

# Egg and Brandy Hair Revitalizer

*For this recipe, I recommend using inexpensive French brandy or cognac, which works to stimulate hair roots and improve circulation in the scalp, thus making your hair look fuller and stronger. Eggs nourish the hair with proteins and fats so that hair looks shiny and smooth. Essential oils help mask the strong smell of the spirit, which many people find a little unpleasant. But it's of course up to you!*

## Ingredients

2–3 egg yolks, depending on your hair length
3–5 tablespoons brandy or cognac
1 tablespoon caster sugar
10 drops geranium essential oil (optional)
5 drops lemon essential oil (optional)

## Method

Whisk egg yolks with cognac, adding just enough caster sugar to make a thicker paste. Add essential oils, if using, and stir well.

## Application

Apply the mask to dry, unwashed hair. Cover your head with a shower cap and wrap it with a towel. Leave the mask on for twenty minutes or more. Rinse off and follow with a mild shampoo.

## Storage

This mask cannot be stored and should be used on the day of preparation.

# Spicy Lemon Anti-Dandruff Shampoo

*This shampoo contains a proven anti-bacterial and anti-inflammatory blend used in Petite Marie Organics SKINSAVER moisturizers for acne-prone skin. You can use Castile soap to make this shampoo; otherwise, you can use a Basic Cleanser recipe from the Cleansing chapter. Make this shampoo in a large batch and give a bottle to everyone you know who may suffer from dandruff. It is very inexpensive and easy to make, and it works miracles. If you want your shampoo to make a lot of foam, add ½ teaspoon decyl glucoside (for sources, see Appendix A)*

## Ingredients

3 oz Castile soap
1 tablespoon glycerin (if using Castile soap)
1 teaspoon jojoba oil (if using Castile soap)
3 tablespoons witch hazel
1 teaspoon marigold (calendula) macerated oil
20 drops tea tree oil
10 drops clove essential oil
8 drops lemon grass essential oil
7 drops eucalyptus essential oil
½ teaspoon zinc oxide

## Method

Prepare the Basic Cleanser according to the recipe in the Cleansing chapter. If using Castile soap, soften it with glycerin and jojoba oil; stir well. Gradually add the remaining ingredients. To help dissolve zinc oxide, add a tablespoon of cleanser or witch hazel, make a smooth paste, and then add to the remaining ingredients. Stir well. Transfer to a plastic or glass bottles. If you need more shampoo, simply multiply the recipe.

## Application

Every day, massage a small amount into wet hair, leave it on for one minute, and then rinse off. Please note that this shampoo is loaded with natural ingredients, so it will not foam lavishly.

## Storage

Store up to nine months in a closed container. Please replace the lid promptly after use.

# Lemon and Vinegar Shine Booster

*Lemon is such a great multitasker! Not only does it helps revive blonde hair, but it also helps impart gorgeous shine to all shades and types of hair. Vinegar is a traditional hair rinse, and geranium distillate helps boost circulation in the scalp for stronger, healthier hair.*

## Ingredients

3 cups apple cider or white wine vinegar
1 lemon
3 cups geranium distillate

## Method

Pour the vinegar into a wide-neck glass bottle. Chop the lemon with its skin on. Add lemon to the vinegar and close the bottle. Leave in a warm place for one to two days, shaking occasionally. Strain the liquid and discard the lemon pieces. Pour the fragrant vinegar into a spray bottle. Add geranium distillate and shake well.

## Application

To use, mist evenly on towel-dried hair, leave on for two to three minutes, and rinse with lukewarm water.

## Storage

Store up to six months in a glass or polypropylene container.

# Grape and Clay Hair Volumizing Treatment

*Clay helps remove excess oils that often result in limp, dull-looking hair. Grapes feed the scalp with antioxidants, while helping to gently polish away dead skin cells. Healthy, shiny, bouncy hair can emerge only from a healthy scalp. Keep that in mind!*

## Ingredients

2–3 cups grape juice (any variety)
1 tablespoon white clay
1 cup green tea
2 tablespoons apple cider vinegar

## Method

Combine all ingredients in a glass or polypropylene (PP) bottle and shake well.

## Application

Shampoo your hair as usual. Pour liberally over wet hair and massage lightly into scalp and along your hair length. Allow to remain on your hair for one minute or more, and then rinse off with cool water. Towel dry your hair and style as usual.

## Storage

This blend can be stored up to one week in a cold, clean place, ideally in a refrigerator.

# Bath Treatment

A bath is more than a simple body-cleansing ritual. It's your chance to relax profoundly, steam your face, and nourish your skin with warm oils that lock the water in your skin, thus delivering triple moisturizing benefits. Your bath can be deeply cleansing, energizing, relaxing, soothing, and even promote weight loss. There are so many simple natural ingredients to add to your bath water, you can mix and match them to suit your skin condition and mood. Here are some kitchen staples to add to your bath:

Milk and cream
Soy, almond, rice milk drinks
Dry dairy and soy milk powder
Almond and oat meal
Sea and Epsom salt
Baking soda
Green tea
Chamomile tea and dried flowers
Peppermint tea and fresh leaves
Vegetable and nut oils
Oranges and lemons
Apple cider vinegar
Fruit juices

# Aromatic Bath Vinegar

*Apple cider vinegar has lots of beauty uses, but when you add it to bath water, it helps tone and firm the skin, relieve dryness, remove skin flakiness, and even soothe itchiness and rashes. Look for dark vinegar, possibly with some residue, which is harmless and actually contains even higher amounts of phytonutrients as compared to transparent light vinegars. You can use all three herbs in equal proportions.*

## Ingredients

4 cups apple cider vinegar
4 cups green tea prepared from 4 tea sachets
5 tablespoons fresh rosemary, peppermint, or lavender
4 drops lemon verbena essential oil
5 drops geranium essential oil
3 drops lavender essential oil
3 drops neroli essential oil

## Method

Steep four packets of green tea in boiling water. Cover and set aside. Crush the herbs of your choice, using pestle and mortar. Pour the vinegar into a large bottle, add the herbs and the tea. Shake well until herbs are thoroughly coated with liquid. Close tightly and store in a dark place.

## Application

Add one cup of fragrant vinegar to your bath water.

## Storage

Store up to three months in a cool, dark place.

# Lemon Foaming Shower Clay

*Rhassoul mud is a natural foaming clay with wonderful skin detox-ifying properties. Unlike conventional detergents, it is not drying and can be used to cleanse your body from head to toes, even if you are prone to dry skin, eczema, or dermatitis. Soothing, naturally anti-bacterial honey is combined with moisturizing aloe vera, while lemon and orange revive your senses. Feel free to experiment with other citrus oils to find a combination that suits your skin (and your nose) best.*

## Ingredients

1 cup filtered tap water
3 cups rhassoul mud
3 tablespoons runny honey
½ cup aloe vera juice
10 drops orange essential oil
10 drops lemon essential oil
½ teaspoon vitamin E oil (as a preservative)

## Method

Combine the ingredients in a non-metal bowl and give it a good stir. Transfer to a glass or plastic jar or a bottle.

## Application

Use as much as required to shampoo your hair or to shower.

## Storage

Store up to three months in a closed container.

# Flower Bath Salts

*Rose and lavender is a classic relaxing luxurious combination, and baking soda helps soften hard water and soothe your skin. By adding a few drops of lemon balm and chamomile, you will help relieve any skin rashes and irritations (do not add chamomile if you are allergic to flowers in the ragweed family). Jasmine oil is quite expensive, but it adds a gorgeous fragrance to this blend.*

## Ingredients

1 cup baking soda
2 cups sea salt
5 drops rose essential oil
5 drops lavender essential oil
5 drops chamomile, jasmine, or lemon balm essential oil

## Method

Place the salt and baking soda in a jar, mason jars are good for this purpose, and shake well to blend. Drizzle essential oils on top of the mixture. Close the lid tightly and shake well. Keep tightly closed until ready to use.

## Application

Dissolve ¼ cup of the salts in your bath water. Allow the salts to dissolve completely before entering the bath.

## Storage

Store up to twelve months in a tightly closed container.

# Aphrodisiac Bath Infusion

*The Indian tradition of Ayurveda recommends that women should wear jasmine on their hands, patchouli on their necks, musk on the abdomen, sandalwood on the thighs, saffron on their feet, and amber on their breasts. This sensual bath infusion may help invigorate libido and revive passion in both men and women.*

## Ingredients

> 1 dried saffron stem
> 1 cup grape seed oil
> 2 teaspoons sucrose laurate or another oil-soluble emulsifier
> 20 drops patchouli essential oil
> 12 drops sandalwood essential oil
> 8 drops jasmine essential oil

## Method

Place the saffron into an empty glass bottle. Fill the bottle with oil and add the emulsifier of your choice. Add essential oils. Shake well and leave to infuse for one day.

## Application

To use, add three to four tablespoons under running warm water to prepare a fragrant, milky bath. To use as a body oil or massage oil, remove the emulsifier from the formulation.

## Storage

Store up to eighteen months in a closed dark glass container.

# Orange Flower Bath Oil

*Bath oils moisturize your skin by floating on the water surface and adhering to your skin as you emerge or splash in the bath. Essential oils evaporate off the warm water surface and penetrate your skin and enter your body as you breathe.*

## Ingredients

1 oz grape seed oil
10 drops orange blossom (neroli) oil
10 drops mandarin essential oil
5 drops bergamot essential oil
5 drops jasmine essential oil
1 tablespoon honey

## Method

Combine all ingredients in a glass container and shake or stir well.

## Application

Use two to three tablespoons per bath. Add to the running water and stir to disperse.

## Storage

Store up to twelve months in a tightly closed container. Close the lid well after each use.

# Sensual Relaxing Bath Oil

*Hippocrates recommended the use of scented oils in the bath, and in ancient Greece balms made with thyme, sage, anise, mint, rose, iris, and marjoram were quite popular. This bath oil can also be used for sensual massage. It makes a wonderful Valentine's Day gift for any romantic soul.*

## Ingredients

3.3 oz apricot kernel or sweet almond oil
20 drops ylang ylang essential oil
10 drops patchouli essential oil
10 drops petitgrain essential oil
5 drops jasmine essential oil

## Method

Combine all ingredients in a dark glass bottle and shake well.

## Application

Add two to three tablespoons under running water to prepare a bath. Use sparingly for body massage.

## Storage

Store up to eighteen months in a tightly closed container away from heat and sunlight. Close the container tightly after each use to prevent essential oils from evaporating or going rancid.

# Invigorating Bath Salt

*I recommend using coarse sea salt for bath salts because it is less expensive, yet holds fragrance just as well as fine salt. Baking soda (sodium bicarbonate) softens the water and soothes the skin. If you want to make more of this salt, multiply the recipe.*

## Ingredients

3 cups coarse sea salt
½ cup baking soda
20 drops geranium essential oil
20 drops neroli essential oil
10 drops mandarin essential oil
5 drops benzoin essential oil (optional)
5 drops jasmine essential oil (optional)

## Method

Combine the salt and baking soda in a glass jar. Add essential oils and stir well to distribute the oils evenly. Close the jar and shake more. Leave the mixture to infuse for 24 hours, and then shake again. The salt is ready to use.

## Application

Add half a cup of salt to the bath water. Stir well.

## Storage

Store up to twelve months in a closed container. Close the lid promptly after each use.

# Calming Chamomile Bath Infusion

*This recipe is based on a traditional European bath preparation for newborns. Chamomile is rich in a natural soothing phytochemical bisabolol that can be very helpful if you suffer from dermatitis, sunburns, or other skin ailments. You can buy whole dried chamomile flowers in health food stores or online (see Appendix A for sources). Alternatively, you can use chamomile tea bags. Any kind of chamomile can be used for the bath.*

## Ingredients

2 cups water
1 cup dried chamomile flowers or 8 chamomile tea bags
3 green tea bags
½ cup dried birch leaves (optional)
½ cup nettle leaves or 4 nettle tea bags

## Method

Combine all ingredients (loose herbs or tea bags if using) in a non-metal bowl or a sauce pan. Pour boiling water on top and let steep for 30 minutes. Alternatively, cover all ingredients with cold water and simmer on low heat for fifteen minutes. Let cool down and strain through cheese cloth. Discard the herbs and store the infusion in a tightly closed container.

## Application

Add 2 cups infusion to the bath water.

## Storage

Store chilled for up to 10 days. Discard if mold forms on the surface.

# Anti Cellulite Bath Salt

*This bath salt relieves water retention, which helps smooth and even skin texture. Epsom salts are very relaxing and may help you unwind after vigorous exercise. It can also be used as a base for a body scrub. Feel free to multiply the recipe if needed.*

## Ingredients

2 cups sea salt
1 cup Epsom salt
½ cup baking soda
20 drops grapefruit essential oil
20 drops pine essential oil
10 drops black pepper essential oil
10 drops mandarin essential oil

## Method

Combine the salt and baking soda in a glass jar. Add essential oils and stir well to distribute the oils evenly. Close the jar and shake more. Leave the mixture to infuse for 24 hours, and then shake again. The salt is ready to use.

## Application

Add half a cup of salt to the bath water. Stir well. To make a body exfoliating treatment for use on thighs and other problem areas, blend one tablespoon salt with three tablespoons plant or nut oil of your choice.

## Storage

Store up to twelve months in a closed container. Close the lid promptly after using the salt.

# Purifying Skin Soak

*This is an astringent, purifying bath preparation that may help diminish body acne and other skin imperfections. Essential oils will not disperse in clay, so we will prepare a creamy mixture that can be used for homemade body clay wraps.*

## Ingredients

3 cups / 0.5 lb green clay
2 green tea bags
2 cups mineral water
2 tablespoons sea salt
3 tablespoons glycerin
20 drops clove essential oil
20 drops tea tree essential oil
15 drops lemon grass essential oil
1 teaspoon calendula macerated oil

## Method

Place the clay and salt into the glass jar. Prepare the green tea by placing the tea bags into boiled mineral water. Steep the tea and discard the bags. Carefully pour the tea into the clay and salt mixture. Stir well to avoid lumps. Add glycerin and stir more. Add essential oils and continue stirring. Adjust the thickness by adding more green tea or water.

## Application

Dissolve four to five tablespoon of clay mixture under running water. To use as a body wrap, apply a thin layer on problem areas and cover with plastic film. Leave on for ten to fifteen minutes or longer, if your skin tolerates it well, then rinse with tepid water.

## Storage

Store up to one month in a closed container, possibly chilled.

# 2-in-1 Slimming Body Scrub and Wrap

*Coffee helps skin lose excess water, thus promoting smooth and even texture, while coffee granules gently exfoliate and nourish the skin with the antioxidant phytochemicals in coffee bean. This scrub smells amazing by itself, but you can also add some skin-tightening citrus oils for maximum skin-toning effects without any expensive synthetic creams. This scrub is featured in my book, Tummy Tuck Diet. This recipe makes one application of the scrub.*

## Ingredients

5 tablespoons ground coffee
2 tablespoons fine salt
½ cup orange juice
1 tablespoon glycerin
1 tablespoon corn flour
5 drops grapefruit essential oil
5 drops lemon/mandarin essential oil
PVC-free plastic film or wide elastic bandages
A blanket or a throw

## Method

Combine the coffee, salt, corn flour, and orange juice in a bowl and stir well to make a smooth sticky paste. Add essential oils if using and stir well.

## Application

Apply the scrub with your fingertips using circular movements. Massage your skin for one to two minutes, and then cover the treated areas with PVC-free plastic film or elastic bandages. Relax for twenty to twenty-five minutes. For maximum effect, cover the treated areas with a throw or a blanket. Make sure to drink lots of fluids with this water-purging skin treatment.

## Storage

This treatment must ideally be used on the day of preparation. However, if you want to enjoy very visible results, you may want to try this treatment every day for five or seven days.

# Inch Loss Clay Body Wrap

*I make this wrap every day for seven days before each swimsuit season. While I treat only my waist and belly area, this wrap works equally well on thighs and other flabby, dimpled areas that could use some serious tightening and lifting. This recipe makes enough clay mixture for one treatment of belly and thigh area. Feel free to multiply the recipe depending on your needs.*

## Ingredients

5 cups / 1lb / 500mg white clay
1 tablespoon ground turmeric
½ teaspoon ground pepper
1 teaspoon spirulina powder (optional)
1 teaspoon ground ginger (optional)
2–3 cups water
2–3 wide elastic or gauze bandages
Old large towels or a blanket

## Method

Place the clay and spices in a bowl and stir well. Carefully add water to make a thin paste.

## Application

Place the bandages into the clay mixture and make sure they are completely saturated and covered with clay. Apply the bandages onto dry skin and wrap them evenly in mummy-like fashion. Secure the ends of bandages with safety pins. Cover a sofa with an old towel and relax for twenty to thirty minutes. Cover yourself with a blanket to keep the treated areas warm, but do not cover them with plastic film. Make sure to drink lots of fluids, because this treatment encourages rapid water loss. After the treatment, rinse the clay with tepid water.

TIP: Emergency blankets made of foil-lined plastic film can be used to cover the treated areas. They conserve your body heat. Extra warmth will ensure even more efficient loss of excess water and promote lymph drainage.

## Storage

Premixed clay and spices can be stored for up to 1 year in an air-tight container.

# 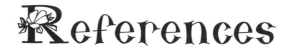References

The following are the major resources used in writing this book.

Djokić, S. "Synthesis and antimicrobial activity of silver citrate complexes," *Bioinorganic Chemistry and Applications*, 2008:436–458.

Hussain, S; Thomassen, LC; Ferecatu, I; Borot, MC; Andreau, K; Martens, JA; Fleury, J; Baeza-Squiban, A; Marano, F; Boland, S. "Carbon black and titanium dioxide nanoparticles elicit distinct apoptotic pathways in bronchial epithelial cells," *Particle and Fibre Toxicology,* 2010 Apr 16:7–10.

Trouiller, B; Reliene, R; Westbrook, A; Solaimani, P; Schiestl, RH. "Titanium dioxide nanoparticles induce DNA damage and genetic instability in vivo in mice," *Cancer Research*, 2009 Nov 15;69(22):8784–9.

## Metric Conversion Chart

Volume Equivalents

1/4 teaspoon=1 ml

1/2 teaspoon=2 ml

1 teaspoon=5 ml

1 tablespoon=15 ml

1/4 cup=50 ml

1/3 cup=75 ml

1/2 cup=125 ml

2/3 cup=150 ml

3/4 cup=175 ml

1 cup=250 ml

1 quart=1 liter= 1000 ml

1-1/2 quarts=1.5 liters

2 quarts=2 liters


Weight Equivalents

1/2 ounce=14 grams

1 ounce=28 grams

2 ounces=56 grams

3 ounces=85 grams

4 ounces=1/4 pound =115 grams

8 ounces=1/2 pound=225 grams

16 ounces=1 pound=455 grams

# 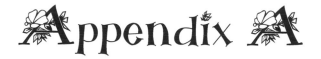Appendix A

## Where to Buy Natural Ingredients

I love researching new ingredients and working with small-scale suppliers of essential oils, herbs, and teas. I have found lots of new exciting ingredients online, at **eBay** (www.ebay.com), in local groceries, health food stores, and pharmacies. Sea salt, sugar, oils, and spices can be purchased inexpensively at your local grocery store or a supermarket.

**Mountain Rose Herbs** (www.mountainroseherbs.com) is one of the oldest and most reputable suppliers of herbs, hydrosols, waxes, essential oils, clays, vegetable glycerin, plant oils and butters, and organic Castile soap for the cosmetic DIY community. In fact, you can find most of the ingredients mentioned in this book at Mountain Rose Herbs. Their shipping prices (even worldwide) are reasonable and customer service is friendly and knowledgeable. Mountain Rose Herbs is a certified organic processor through Oregon Tilth.

**Ingredients to Die For** (www.ingredientstodiefor.com) is a great source of high-end active ingredients, such as allantoin, salicylic acid, royal jelly, ascorbyl palmitate (vitamin C ester), alpha lipoic acid, and resveratrol. You will also find a selection of ready-made products, many of which contain no harmful preservatives, and a wide range of natural and safe semi-natural emulsifiers, thickeners, surfactants, penetration enhancers, and stabilizers for a serious cosmetic formulator.

**Texas Natural Supply** (www.texasnaturalsupply.com) sells amazing base products made entirely without synthetic chemicals and suitable for many hard-to-deal-with skin conditions. This store has a vast selection of clays, powders, surfactants, and preservatives, including silver citrate. I recommend visiting a tool section that offers indispensable pH test strips, pipettes, masks, self-sealing bags, and medical beakers.

**Skin Actives** (www.skinactives.com). Dr. Hanna Sivak and Jonatan Funtowicz were the first to offer ready-to-use sophisticated active ingredients normally found in high-end department store lines. Head on to this Web site for hard-to-find, powerful peptides and antioxidants, such as phloretin, açaí, argireline, ellagic acid, copper peptides, adenosine triphosphate, resveratrol, and coffee essential oil. These skincare gems will arrive in cute little tubes along with instruction for use and spatulas for mixing your actives into your favorite homemade or store-bought cream.

**Camden-Grey** (www.camdengrey.com) has an amazing selection of oils and butters, beeswax in blocks and easy-to-melt pearls, aloe in gels, powders, and juice, and very useful preservatives, such as all-natural vitamin E and grapefruit seed extract. I recommend trying açaí butter, wild-crafted Castile soap, and colored jojoba beads to give your homemade scrubs a touch of spa glamour.

**Making Cosmetics** (www.makingcosmetics.com) is an information-packed online store selling an amazing selection of ready-made bases for an advanced DIY beauty enthusiast. I recommend trying liquid vitamin C, rice peptides, organic colors for your makeup creations, liposomes, and body odor neutralizing zinc ricinoleate for your homemade deodorants.

**Essentially Oils** (www.essentiallyoils.co.uk) is a UK-based supplier of inexpensive essential oils, organic flower waters and hydrosols, oils and butters, as well as reasonably priced glass and plastic bottles and jars.

## Where to Buy Cosmetic Packaging

**Freeman and Harding** (www.freemanharding.co.uk) offers a great range of inexpensive glass oil bottles and plastic tubs suitable for both large producers of aromatherapy oils and small-scale DIY beauty enthusiasts.

# 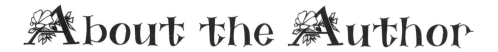 About the Author

Julie Gabriel is a holistic nutritionist educated at the Canadian School of Natural Nutrition. A former magazine beauty editor, a television journalist, a weight loss coach, and a committed green mom, Julie Gabriel is a dedicated green living and holistic natural eating. Julie has been featured on Martha Stewart's Living Radio, in *USA Today, The Washington Post, Toronto Star, Sun Sentinel, Natural Solutions, Body & Soul*, and many other publications.

At Julie Gabriel's Web site, you will find the latest news and features on diet, nutrition, weight loss, organic eating and lifestyle, and many much more.

You can explore Julie's publications, read reviews, and download books and free eBooks.

Every month, a lucky subscriber to the BEAUTY FULL LIFE newsletter wins an organic beauty product by Petite Marie Organics or one of the carefully selected organic and natural beauty brands.

Follow the BEAUTY FULL LIFE newsletter on Twitter (holistic-beauty, twitnutrition) or become a subscriber yourself at www.juliegabriel.com.

## Books by Julie Gabriel

CLEAR SKIN: Organic Action Plan for Acne (iUniverse 2007)

THE GREEN BEAUTY GUIDE: Your Essential Resource to Organic and Natural Skincare, Haircare, Makeup and Fragrances (HCI, 2008)

GREEN BEAUTY RECIPES: 300 Easy All-Natural Recipes to Make Your Own Natural Skincare, Hair Care, and Body Care Products (Petite Marie Publishing, 2010)

THE LIBIDO DIET: The Holistic Nutritional Plan to Revitalize your Love Life, Restore your Sexual Wellbeing, and Rejuvenate your Body and Mind (Petite Marie Books, February 2011)

VEGAN BEAUTY RECIPES: Animal-Free, Plant-Based Recipes to Make Your Own Natural Skincare, Hair Care, Anti Aging and Skin Rejuvenation Products (April 2011, Petite Marie Books)

THE TUMMY TUCK DIET: The Holistic System to Achieve a Sexy Flat Yummy Tummy and Lose Toxic Belly Fat (Petite Marie Publishing, June 2011)

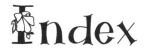

# Index

Olive

    *Leaf extract*, 82, 86

    *Oil*, 21, 46, 60, 71, 80, 83, 86, 95, 103, 106, 125, 127, 137, 149, 155, 169, 171, 191, 205

Orange

    *Essential oil*, 169, 207, 215, 218

    *Fruit*, 32, 94, 213

    *Juice*, 66, 108, 152, 225

    *Water*, 41, 87, 192

Oregano essential oil, 26

**P**

Panthenol (pro-vitamin B5), 77

Papaya, 21, 54, 68, 108, 114

Parabens, 23

Patch test, 4

Patchouli essential oil, 166, 167, 168, 169, 171, 217, 219

Peach, 51

Peppermint

    *Essential oil*, 84, 94, 147, 186, 193

    *Herb*, 116, 188, 199, 213, 214

Petroleum, 3

Phenoxyethanol, 21

Pine essential oil, 222

Polyethylene terephthalate (PET), 27

Polypropylene, 26

Polysorbate, 18

Pomegranate, 66

Potassium sorbate, 24

Potato, 13, 66, 108, 125, 130, 131, 139, 140, 204

Poultice, 13

Pumpkin

    *Fruit*, 118, 124

    *Seed oil*, 21

**R**

Rhassoul clay, 37, 215

Rose

    *Essential oil*, 26, 40, 80, 91, 96, 106, 112, 149, 150, 157, 160, 169, 181, 202, 205, 216

    *Petals*, 80, 171

    *Water*, 58, 80, 89, 109, 165, 167

Rosehip oil, 21, 84, 95

Rosemary

    *Fresh*, 64, 214

    *Essential oil*, 26, 89, 109, 165, 167

    *Extract*, 25, 41, 63

**S**

Sage essential oil, 26

Sake, 64

Salt, 32, 33, 51, 100, 120, 126, 133,

Made in the USA
San Bernardino, CA
03 March 2014